Ending the War against Children: the Rights of Children to Live Free of Violence

Editors

DANIELLE LARAQUE-ARENA
BONITA F. STANTON

PEDIATRIC CLINICS OF NORTH AMERICA

www.pediatric.theclinics.com

Consulting Editor
BONITA F. STANTON

April 2021 • Volume 68 • Number 2

ELSEVIER

1600 John F. Kennedy Boulevard • Suite 1800 • Philadelphia, Pennsylvania, 19103-2899

http://www.theclinics.com

THE PEDIATRIC CLINICS OF NORTH AMERICA Volume 68, Number 2
April 2021 ISSN 0031-3955, ISBN-13: 978-0-323-83610-4

Editor: Kerry Holland
Developmental Editor: Axell Ivan Jade M. Purificacion

The Pediatric Clinics of North America (ISSN 0031-3955) is published bimonthly by Elsevier Inc., 360 Park Avenue South, New York, NY 10010-1710. Months of issue are February, April, June, August, October, and December. Periodicals postage paid at New York, NY and additional mailing offices. Subscription prices are $250.00 per year (US individuals), $984.00 per year (US institutions), $315.00 per year (Canadian individuals), $1048.00 per year (Canadian institutions), $376.00 per year (international individuals), $1048.00 per year (international institutions), $100.00 per year (US students and residents), $100.00 per year (Canadian students and residents), and $165.00 per year (international residents and students). To receive students/resident rare, orders must be accompanied by name of affiliated institution, date of term, and the signature of program/residency coordinator on institution letterhead. Orders will be billed at individual rate until proof of status is received. Foreign air speed delivery is included in all *Clinics* subscription prices. All prices are subject to change without notice. **POSTMASTER:** Send address changes to *The Pediatric Clinics of North America*, Elsevier Health Sciences Division, Subscription Customer Service, 3251 Riverport Lane, Maryland Heights, MO 63043. **Customer Service: 1-800-654-2452 (US and Canada). From outside of the US and Canada: 1-314-447-8871. Fax: 1-314-447-8029. For print support, E-mail: JournalsCustomerService-usa@elsevier.com. For online support, E-mail: JournalsOnlineSupport-usa@elsevier.com.**

Reprints. For copies of 100 or more, of articles in this publication, please contact the Commercial Reprints Department, Elsevier Inc., 360 Park Avenue South, New York, NY 10010-1710. Tel.: 212-633-3874; Fax: 212-633-3820; E-mail: reprints@elsevier.com.

The Pediatric Clinics of North America is also published in Spanish by McGraw-Hill Inter-americana Editores S.A., Mexico City, Mexico; in Portuguese by Riechmann and Affonso Editores, Rua Comandante Coelho 1085, CEP 21250, Rio de Janeiro, Brazil; and in Greek by Althayia SA, Athens, Greece.

The Pediatric Clinics of North America is covered in *MEDLINE/PubMed (Index Medicus), Excerpta Medica, Current Contents, Current Contents/Clinical Medicine, Science Citation Index, ASCA, ISI/BIOMED*, and *BIOSIS*.

Printed in the United States of America.

PROGRAM OBJECTIVE
The goal of the *Pediatric Clinics of North America* is to keep practicing physicians and residents up to date with current clinical practice in pediatrics by providing timely articles reviewing the state-of-the-art in patient care.

TARGET AUDIENCE
All practicing pediatricians, physicians and healthcare professionals who provide patient care to pediatric patients.

LEARNING OBJECTIVES
Upon completion of this activity, participants will be able to:
1. Review the epidemiology and global burden of disease from violent acts against children.
2. Discuss forcible displacement, firearm injuries in urban areas, rural communities and violence, attacks on schools and other public spaces, sexual violence against children inclusive of abduction, trafficking, intrafamilial abuse and child marriage, war, conflict and terrorism, racism and other systems of structural inequities as violence against children, the impact of intimate partner violence, and executions and police conflicts.
3. Recognize evidence-based interventions to reduce violence to children and brings in the perspective of clinical care, education, research and policy imperatives.

ACCREDITATIONS
Physician Credit

The Elsevier Office of Continuing Medical Education (EOCME) is accredited by the Accreditation Council for Continuing Medical Education (ACCME) to provide continuing medical education for physicians.

The EOCME designates this journal-based activity for a maximum of 13 *AMA PRA Category 1 Credit*(s)™. Physicians should claim only the credit commensurate with the extent of their participation in the activity.

All other healthcare professionals requesting continuing education credit for this this journal-based activity will be issued a certificate of participation.

ABP Maintenance of Certification Credit

Successful completion of this CME activity, which includes participation in the activity and individual assessment of and feedback to the learner, enables the learner to earn up to 13 MOC points in the American Board of Pediatrics' (ABP) Maintenance of Certification (MOC) program. It is the CME activity provider's responsibility to submit learner completion information to ACCME for the purpose of granting ABP MOC credit.

DISCLOSURE OF CONFLICTS OF INTEREST
The EOCME assesses conflict of interest with its instructors, faculty, planners, and other individuals who are in a position to control the content of CME activities. All relevant conflicts of interest that are identified are thoroughly vetted by EOCME for fair balance, scientific objectivity, and patient care recommendations. EOCME is committed to providing its learners with CME activities that promote improvements or quality in healthcare and not a specific proprietary business or a commercial interest.

The planning committee, staff, authors, and editors listed below have identified no financial relationships or relationships to products or devices they or their spouse/life partner have with commercial interest related to the content of this CME activity:
Miriam Abaya, JD; Nina Agrawal; Charles C. Branas, PhD; Shaelyn M. Cavanaugh, MPH; Diego Chaves-Gnecco, MD, MPH, FAAP; Regina Chavous-Gibson, MSN, RN; Brittney Davis, MPH; James M. Dodington, MD; Ruth A. Etzel, MD, PhD; Glenn Flores, MD, FAAP; Margaret K. Formica, MSPH, PhD; Ariana Gobaud, MPH; Jeffrey Goldhagen, MD; Kerry Holland; Gillian Hopgood, DO, FAAP; Tiffani J. Johnson, MD, MSc; Camara Phyllis Jones, MD, MPH, PhD; Danielle Laraque-Arena, MD, FAAP; Lori Legano, MD, FAAP; Bruce Lesley; Rajkumar Mayakrishnann; Madeline Mineo; Rita Nathawad, MD; Kathleen O'Neill, MD, MPH; Charles Oberg, MD; Sonali Rajan, EdD; Shanti Raman, PhD; Paul M. Reeping, MS; Bonita Stanton, MD; Luisa Vaca Condado; Ingrid Walker-Descartes, MD, MPH, MBA, FAAP; Claire Williams; Joseph L. Wright, MD, MPH.

UNAPPROVED/OFF-LABEL USE DISCLOSURE
The EOCME requires CME faculty to disclose to the participants:
1. When products or procedures being discussed are off-label, unlabelled, experimental, and/or investigational (not US Food and Drug Administration [FDA] approved); and

2. Any limitations on the information presented, such as data that are preliminary or that represent ongoing research, interim analyses, and/or unsupported opinions. Faculty may discuss information about pharmaceutical agents that is outside of FDA-approved labelling. This information is intended solely for CME and is not intended to promote off-label use of these medications. If you have any questions, contact the medical affairs department of the manufacturer for the most recent prescribing information.

TO ENROLL

To enroll in the *Pediatric Clinics of North America* Continuing Medical Education program, call customer service at 1-800-654-2452 or sign up online at http://www.theclinics.com/home/cme. The CME program is available to subscribers for an additional annual fee of USD 324.00.

METHOD OF PARTICIPATION

In order to claim credit, participants must complete the following:
1. Complete enrolment as indicated above.
2. Read the activity.
3. Complete the CME Test and Evaluation. Participants must achieve a score of 70% on the test. All CME Tests and Evaluations must be completed online.

In order to claim MOC points, participants must complete the following:
1. Complete steps listed above for claiming CME credit
2. Provide your specialty board ID#, birth date (MM/DD), and attestation.
3. Online MOC submission is only available for the American Board of pediatrics' (ABP) Maintenance of Certification (MOC) program

CME INQUIRIES/SPECIAL NEEDS

For all CME inquiries or special needs, please contact elsevierCME@elsevier.com.

Contributors

CONSULTING EDITOR

BONITA F. STANTON, MD
Founding Dean, Robert C. and Laura C. Garrett Endowed Chair, Hackensack Meridian
School of Medicine, President, Academic Enterprise, Hackensack Meridian Health,
Nutley, New Jersey, USA

EDITORS

DANIELLE LARAQUE-ARENA, MD, FAAP
Senior Scholar in Residence, New York Academy of Medicine, Adjunct Professor of
Epidemiology, Columbia University Mailman School of Public Health, Associate Director
Injury Free Coalition for Kids, National Program, New York, New York, USA; President and
Professor Emerita, SUNY Upstate Medical University, Syracuse, New York, USA

BONITA F. STANTON, MD
Founding Dean, Robert C. and Laura C. Garrett Endowed Chair, Hackensack Meridian
School of Medicine, President, Academic Enterprise, Hackensack Meridian Health,
Nutley, New Jersey, USA

AUTHORS

MIRIAM ABAYA, JD
Senior Director, Immigration and Children's Rights, First Focus on Children, Washington,
DC, USA

NINA AGRAWAL, MD, FAAP
Child Abuse Pediatrician and Masters Candidate, City University of New York (CUNY)
School of Public Health, New York, New York, USA

CHARLES C. BRANAS, PhD
Gelman Endowed Professor, Department of Epidemiology, Columbia University Mailman
School of Public Health, New York, New York, USA

SHAELYN M. CAVANAUGH, MPH
Department of Public Health and Preventive Medicine, SUNY Upstate Medical University,
Syracuse, New York, USA

DIEGO CHAVES-GNECCO, MD, MPH, FAAP
Program Director and Founder, Salud Para Niños Program, UPMC Children's Hospital of
Pittsburgh, Associate Professor, Department of Pediatrics, University of Pittsburgh School
of Medicine, Pittsburgh, Pennsylvania, USA

LUISA VACA CONDADO, BA
Coordinator - Fellowship and Research Programs, Department of Pediatrics, Maimonides
Children's Hospital of Brooklyn, Brooklyn, New York, USA

BRITTNEY DAVIS, MPH
New York Academy of Medicine, New York, New York, USA

JAMES M. DODINGTON, MD
Assistant Professor of Pediatrics and Emergency Medicine, Yale School of Medicine, New Haven, Connecticut, USA

RUTH A. ETZEL, MD, PhD
Adjunct Professor, Department of Environmental and Occupational Health, Milken Institute School of Public Health, The George Washington University, Washington, DC, USA

GLENN FLORES, MD, FAAP
Professor and Chair of Pediatrics, Senior Associate Dean of Child Health, George E. Batchelor Endowed Chair in Child Health, Department of Pediatrics, University of Miami Miller School of Medicine, Physician-in-Chief, Holtz Children's Hospital, Miami, Florida, USA

MARGARET K. FORMICA, MSPH, PhD
Associate Professor, Department of Public Health and Preventive Medicine, SUNY Upstate Medical University, Syracuse, New York, USA

ARIANA N. GOBAUD, MPH
Department of Epidemiology, Columbia University Mailman School of Public Health, New York, New York, USA

JEFFREY GOLDHAGEN, MD
Professor, Department of Pediatrics, Division of Community and Societal Pediatrics, University of Florida, Jacksonville, Florida, USA

GILLIAN HOPGOOD, DO, FAAP
Child Abuse Fellow, Department of Pediatrics, Maimonides Children's Hospital of Brooklyn, Brooklyn, New York, USA

TIFFANI J. JOHNSON, MD, MSc
Assistant Professor of Emergency, Medicine, University of California, Davis School of Medicine, Sacramento, California, USA

CAMARA PHYLLIS JONES, MD, MPH, PhD
Adjunct Professor, Department of Behavioral Sciences and Health Education and Department of Epidemiology, Rollins School of Public Health, Emory University, and Adjunct Associate Professor, Department of Community Health and Preventive Medicine, Morehouse School of Medicine, Atlanta, Georgia, USA

DANIELLE LARAQUE-ARENA, MD, FAAP
Senior Scholar in Residence, New York Academy of Medicine, Adjunct Professor of Epidemiology, Columbia University Mailman School of Public Health, Associate Director, Injury Free Coalition for Kids, National Program, New York, New York, USA; President and Professor Emerita, SUNY Upstate Medical University, Syracuse, New York, USA

LORI LEGANO, MD, FAAP
Director of Child Protection Services, Department of Pediatrics, NYU Grossman School of Medicine, Bellevue Hospital Center, New York, New York, USA

BRUCE LESLEY, BA
President, First Focus on Children, Washington, DC, USA

MADELINE MINEO, DO
Fellow - Child Abuse Pediatrics, Department of Pediatrics, Maimonides Children's
Hospital of Brooklyn, Brooklyn, New York, USA

RITA NATHAWAD, MD
Assistant Professor, Department of Pediatrics, University of Florida, Jacksonville, Florida,
USA

KATHLEEN M. O'NEILL, MD
PhD Candidate, Investigative Medicine Program, Yale School of Medicine, New Haven,
Connecticut, USA

CHARLES OBERG, MD
Professor Emeritus, Global Pediatric Program, University of Minnesota, Minneapolis,
Minnesota, USA

SONALI RAJAN, EdD
Associate Professor of Health Education, Department of Epidemiology, Columbia
University Mailman School of Public Health, Department of Health and Behavior Studies,
Columbia University, Teachers College, New York, New York, USA

SHANTI RAMAN, PhD
Associate Professor, School of Women's and Children's Health, UNSW Sydney, Australia

PAUL M. REEPING, MS
Department of Epidemiology, Columbia University Mailman School of Public Health, New
York, New York, USA

BONITA F. STANTON, MD
Founding Dean, Robert C. and Laura C. Garrett Endowed Chair, Hackensack Meridian
School of Medicine, President, Academic Enterprise, Hackensack Meridian Health,
Nutley, New Jersey, USA

INGRID WALKER-DESCARTES, MD, MPH, MBA, FAAP
Director of Child Maltreatment Services, Department of Pediatrics, Maimonides
Children's Hospital of Brooklyn, Brooklyn, New York, USA

CLAIRE WILLIAMS, BA
Policy Fellow, First Focus on Children, Washington, DC, USA

JOSEPH L. WRIGHT, MD, MPH
Professor of Pediatrics and Health Policy and Management, University of Maryland
Schools of Medicine and Public Health, Cheverly, Maryland, USA

Contents

> In Latin America, violence is a major public health issue causing many fam-
> ilies to flee to the United States to seek safety. Current US immigration pol-
> icies fail to address why families are forced to depart their home country or
> the needs of families once arriving in the United States. This article iden-
> tifies root causes of family displacement, examines the insufficient protec-
> tions for children in families during US immigration processing, and
> provides practice and policy recommendations on how to transform the
> US immigration system so that it is more humane for children and families
> forcibly displaced by violence.

> Firearm violence is a significant public health problem, particularly among
> youth in the United States. Regardless of the data source or setting, young
> Black men have consistently been found to be disproportionately affected
> by firearm injuries and deaths. Public health research indicates that racial
> segregation likely increases racial disparities in firearm violence. To mini-
> mize deaths and injuries due to firearms and their cascading health conse-
> quences and to ultimately achieve health equity, preventive efforts will
> need to address the social determinants of health, including racism.

> Among US geographic regions classified as rural, death rates are signifi-
> cantly higher for children and teens as compared with their urban peers;
> the disparity is even greater for Alaskan Native/American Indian and
> non-Hispanic Black youth. Violence-related injuries and death contribute
> significantly to this finding. This article describes the epidemiology of
> violence-related injuries, with a limited discussion on child abuse and
> neglect and an in-depth analysis of self-inflicted injuries including uninten-
> tional firearm injuries and adolescent suicide. Potential interventions are
> also addressed, including strategies for injury prevention, such as firearm
> safe storage practices.

> Schools should be considered safe spaces for children; children need to
> feel secure in order to grow and learn. This article argues that when a
> school shooting occurs, the harm goes beyond those who are injured or
> killed, because the presumption of security is shattered, and the mental
> and emotional health of the students is threatened. There are many inter-
> ventions for preventing these attacks at the school, state, and federal

levels. This article explores evidence behind some of these interventions and describes the delicate balance in implementing interventions without introducing undue stress and anxiety into a child's everyday life.

Ingrid Walker-Descartes, Gillian Hopgood, Luisa Vaca Condado, and Lori Legano

Sexual violence against children is a gross violation of children's rights during their formative years and will likely interfere with their developmental trajectory and long-term quality of life. This form of violence includes commercial sexual exploitation of children, sexual abuse, child marriages, and female genital mutilation. The evidence shows that violence prevention is worth the investment; however, prioritizing this agenda to ensure funding through government spending remains low. Despite funding realities, research and advocacy efforts need to continue, with a focus on promoting effective practices for mitigation.

Ruth A. Etzel

A child soldier is a person less than 18 years of age who/has been recruited/used by an armed force/armed group in any capacity, including but not limited to children, boys and girls, used as fighters, cooks, porters, messengers, spies, or for sexual purposes. Complex consequences on both physical and mental health are reported among child soldiers. One-third to one-half of these children may have clinically significant symptoms of post-traumatic stress disorder. The United Nations identified more than 25,000 grave violations against children during armed conflicts in 2019. The recruitment and use of children under 18 in armed conflicts must stop.

Camara Phyllis Jones

Racism is a system of structuring opportunity and assigning value based on the social interpretation of how one looks (which is what we call "race"). Racism unfairly disadvantages some individuals and communities, unfairly advantages other individuals and communities, and saps the strength of the whole society through the waste of human resources. There are 7 barriers to achieving health equity that are deeply embedded in US culture. These serve as values targets for anti-racism action. This article is an invitation to all who love children to become actively anti-racism.

Ingrid Walker-Descartes, Madeline Mineo, Luisa Vaca Condado, and Nina Agrawal

Men and women experience severe domestic violence (DV) and intimate partner violence (IPV); however, women and children remain especially vulnerable. Violence along the DV/IPV continuum has been recognized as a type of child maltreatment and a child's awareness that a caregiver is being harmed or at risk of harm is sufficient to induce harmful sequelae. Consequences of these abusive behaviors are associated with mental and physical health consequences. Health care professionals can screen, identify, and manage this pathology in affected families while educating communities to these pernicious effects.

Police violence in the United States represents a pressing public health crisis impacting youth, particularly youth of color. This article reviews the recent epidemiology of police executions and conflicts involving children, adolescents, and young adults. The roles of social determinants of health and centuries-long history of white supremacy and racism as root causes of adverse policing are emphasized. The article summarizes the evidence as to how direct and vicarious experiences of police violence impact youth academic, behavioral, and health outcomes. Recommendations are provided for pediatricians to address this public health crisis through clinical practice, education, advocacy, and research.

Strategies for the prevention of violence against children have evolved over the last 3 decades to incorporate community-engaged approaches. These promising approaches involve mobilizing key stakeholders within communities from a variety of different sectors, and engaging adult bystanders to take action when violence is suspected. However, there are many challenges associated with funding and evaluating such programs, which are often barriers in the development of an evidence base that includes metrics of effectiveness and cost benefits. This article discusses specific interventions developed to target physical abuse and neglect, sexual violence, community and gang violence, and bullying within the community setting.

PEDIATRIC CLINICS OF NORTH AMERICA

SERIES OF RELATED INTEREST

Clinics in Perinatology
http://www.perinatology.theclinics.com/
Advances in Pediatrics
http://www.advancesinpediatrics.com/

THE CLINICS ARE AVAILABLE ONLINE!
Access your subscription at:
www.theclinics.com

Preface

A Twenty-First Century Policy Agenda: Violence in the Lives of Children, Families, and Communities

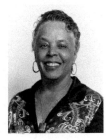 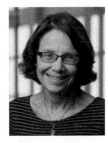

Danielle Laraque-Arena, MD, FAAP   Bonita F. Stanton, MD
Editors

In the twenty-first century, there has been recognition of the substantial progress we have made in the reductions of infant and child morbidity and mortality. Over the period of 1950 to 2017, the under-five mortality rate globally decreased from 216.0 (196.3-238.1) deaths/1000 live births to 38.9 deaths (35.6-42.83)/1000 live births. Nevertheless, 5.4 (5.2-5.6) million deaths among children less than 5 years of age occurred in 2017.[1] In addition, there has been recognition that a much more comprehensive approach is needed to tackle the full scope of what makes today's world uncertain for children despite the progress to date. Issues such as climate change, ecological degradation, migrating populations, conflicts, pervasive inequalities, and predatory commercial practices are threats to the well-being of our children.[2-4] The United Nations Children's Fund (UNICEF) and the World Health Organization (WHO) have categorized child-related indicators of the Sustainable Developmental Goal agenda around 5 dimensions of children's rights: survive and thrive; learning; protection from violence and exploitation; safe and clean environments; and a fair chance at life. This issue of *Pediatric Clinics of North America* focuses the discussion on violence against children in this broad framework as outlined by the WHO and UNICEF.[2] The major persistent, and particularly malignant, issue confronting communities and child health professionals worldwide who wish to improve the lives of children is child trauma as a consequence of acts of violence, whether physical, sexual, psychological, or complex. Furthermore, child trauma, in the context of armed conflict or occurring in or out of the home, cannot and should not be ignored by those interested in local and global child health and mandates an understanding of the broader context of how this

Pediatr Clin N Am 68 (2021) xv–xviii
https://doi.org/10.1016/j.pcl.2021.01.001
0031-3955/21/© 2021 Published by Elsevier Inc.

pediatric.theclinics.com

violence occurs and its root causes. This understanding will offer the hope that comprehensive interventions rather than categorical stopgap measures will address entrenched problems. The approach to elimination of violence against children will require the involvement of diverse disciplines in public health, medicine, and science as well as nonhealth sectors, and the strategies to address violence and exploitation of children will necessarily focus on the 3 central domains of healthy childhood as identified by the WHO-UNICEF[2]: survive (ending preventable deaths), thrive (ensure health and well-being), and transform (expanding enabling environments).

This issue of *Pediatric Clinics of North America* covers a wide range of acts of violence, including the fate of children during armed conflicts. The comprehensive analysis of global armed conflict conducted by the United Nations High Commissioner for Refugees noted that by the end of 2018, 70.8 million individuals were forcibly displaced; one in every 108 people globally is either an asylum-seeker, internally displaced, or a refugee. This is an increase of 2.3 million people over the previous year, and the world's forcibly displaced population remained at a record high. This includes 25.9 million refugees in the world—the highest ever seen; 41.3 million internally displaced people; and 3.5 million asylum-seekers.[5] Children comprised more than half of the refugees, and many were separated from their parents or traveling alone. These displacements bring with them a host of risks for violence against children. In addition, worldwide, the toll of violence against children living in countries with dictatorial regimes, at times exacerbated by drug wars, is reflected in the number of refugees seeking asylum. As the numbers of refugees increase, the willingness of other nations to accept them declines, leaving an ever-increasing portion unable to find asylum other than in temporary, makeshift camps, often with inadequate resources, and leaving children and families even more vulnerable.[5]

The recent Global Burden of Disease Study,[1] 2017 (ghdx.healthdata.org ⟩ gbd-2017), using a new unifying methodology that allows comparisons of injury prevalence and incidence across national boundaries, provides the platform for the discussion of violence of all kinds against children worldwide. Community violence, including that which is the result of penetrating trauma from firearms and stabbings, is a specific external injury cause of morbidity and mortality for children and adolescents worldwide. The number of deaths from small arms (ie, portable arms, such as rifles, handguns, and semiautomatic weapons) mirrors that from declared armed conflicts. For example, in the United States, the cumulative death toll from the Vietnam War was 58,000. However, in 2018, the total number of firearm-related deaths in the United States for all ages was 39,740.[6] That is, every 2 years, civilian lives lost exceed the number of deaths resulting from one of the worst wars in recent US history.[7] Also of great concern, the second - and third - leading causes of death for youth in 2018 were suicide and homicide, respectively, with suicide disproportionately affecting Native American and white male youths and homicide affecting black male youths. Among the top leading violent injuries in 2018 in the United States, homicide unspecified was the leading cause for children 1 to 4 years and homicide firearm for those 5 to 9 years, 10 to 14 years, and 15 to 19 years.[8]

This issue is organized into 3 sections. The first section is an overview of the epidemiology and global burden of disease from violent acts against children. In addition, in this section, we review the rights of children using the framework of the United Nations Conventions on the Rights of the Child, which has called for a worldwide recognition of the rights of children (0-18 years) codified in 54 articles and urging states for worldwide actions to promote the health and well-being of all children.[9] It is notable that in 2020, the United States is the only country in the world to not have ratified the United Nations Conventions on the Rights of the Child. Nonetheless, there is hope in this regard since many activities in the United States have reflected the increasing recognition of the need for clinical, educational, research, and policy efforts within a child rights framework. Examples of such activities include those described by authors using youth participatory principles.[10,11]

It should be noted that there are 232 Sustainable Development Goals indicators, of which 47 relate to child health and well-being.[2] Various sources are used throughout this issue of *Pediatric Clinics of North America* when discussing specific topics that relate to violence against children, and despite our best efforts, there will be data gaps. Most countries are able to report on poverty and health, especially mortality and health care intervention. By contrast, many countries are not prepared to assess newer and less well-established indicators, such as those that relate to gender inequality, particularly important in the discussion of sexual violence. A focus on racial, ethnic, and class-based inequalities is also complicated by the country's particular context and history.

The second section of the issue is organized as case study discussions covering the specific topics of forcible displacement, firearm injuries in urban areas, rural communities and violence, attacks on schools and other public spaces, sexual violence against children inclusive of abduction, trafficking, intrafamilial abuse and child marriage, war, conflict and terrorism, racism and other systems of structural inequities as violence against children, the impact of intimate partner violence, and executions and police conflicts. The categories of violent injuries detailed were guided by the current data report of the Global Health Burden, Lancet Commission.[12] This section covers a broad range of acts of violence against children in order to give the readers a sense of the scope of the problem and the need for comprehensive approaches. The case discussion format conveys, in tangible terms, the human toll of specific forms of violence against children and provides the reader with examples of ways to combat such violence.

The third section reviews the critical literature of evidence-based interventions to reduce violence to children and brings in the perspective of clinical care, education, research, and policy imperatives. The perspective of the Sustainable Development Goals is incorporated in these discussions as well as the broad topic of access to humanitarian support.

This issue of *Pediatric Clinics of North America*, devoted to the subject of the impact of violence on the lives of children worldwide, signals growing collective recognition of the need to address this urgent global problem. We are encouraged that governments across the globe along with countless international, national, and local agencies recognize the needs and rights of children affected by global armed conflict and community violence and their multilayered repercussions. The development of effective interventions to prevent or mitigate violence against children in all its forms is gaining traction. The discussion of child trauma underscores the great significance of the developmental process of childhood and the commitment we must have in addressing the United Nation's Sustainable Development Goal 3 to achieve maximal child health and well-being.[13]

The intended purpose of this issue is to harness the collective wisdom of health professionals knowledgeable in this area to stimulate policy, research, public health, and clinical action to reduce and eventually eliminate violence against children, their families, and communities.

Danielle Laraque-Arena, MD, FAAP
New York Academy of Medicine, 1216 Fifth Avenue
New York, NY 10029, USA

Bonita F. Stanton, MD
Hackensack Meridian School of Medicine
123 Metro Boulevard (formerly 340 Kingsland Street)
Nutley, NJ 07110, USA

E-mail addresses:
Dlaraque-arena@nyam.org (D. Laraque-Arena)
Bonita.Stanton@hackensackmeridian.org (B.F. Stanton)

REFERENCES

1. Global Burden of Disease (GBD) 2017 Mortality Collaborators. Global regional, and national age-sex-specific mortality and life expectancy, 1950-2017: a systematic analysis for the GBD Study 2017. Elsevier; 2018. p. 1684–1735.
2. Clark H, Coll-Seck AW, Banerjee A, et al. A future for the world's children? A WHO-UNICEF-Lancet Commission. Lancet 2020;395(10224):605–58.
3. Laraque D. Global child health: reaching the tipping point for all children. Acad Pediatr 2011;11(3):226–33.
4. Laraque-Arena D, Shahid SH. A new development matrix for global child health. In: Laraque-Arena D, Stanton BF, editors. Principles of global child health: education and research. Itasca (IL): American Academy of Pediatrics; 2019. p. 81–96.
5. Machel G. Available at: gopher://gopher.un.org/00/ga/docs/51/plenary/A51-306. EN. Accessed.
6. Available at: https://www.cdc.gov/injury/wisqars/index.html. Accessed October 20, 2020.
7. Available at: https://www.britannica.com/event/Vietnam-War. Accessed October 20, 2020.
8. Available at: https://webappa.cdc.gov/cgi-bin/broker.exe. Accessed October 20, 2020.
9. United Nations Convention on the Rights of the Child. Available at: https://www.ohchr.org/en/professionalinterest/pages/crc.aspx. Accessed March 17, 2020.
10. Ozer DJ. Youth-Led participatory action research: developmental and equity perspectives. Chapter seven. In: Equity and Justice in Developmental Science: Theoretical and Methodological Issues (SS Horn, MD Ruck & LS Liben, Eds) Advances in Child Development and Behavior (JB Benson, Series Ed) Vol 50 ISSN 0065-2407. Available at: https://dx.doi.org/10.1016/bs.acdb.2015.11.006
11. Hawke LD, Relihan J, Miller J, et al. Engaging youth research in planning, design and execution: practical recommendations for researchers. Health Expect 2018; 21:944–9.
12. GBD 107 Disease and Injury Incidence and Prevalence Collaborators. Global, regional, and national incidence, prevalence, and years lived with disability for 354 diseases and injuries for 195 countries and territories, 1990-2017: a systematic analysis for the Global Burden of Disease Study 2017. Elsevier; 2018. p. 1789–858.
13. Available at: https://www.un.org/sustainabledevelopment/. Accessed.

The War against Children

Global Burden of Violence

Bonita Stanton, MD[a],*, Brittney Davis, MPH[b],
Danielle Laraque-Arena, MD[c]

KEYWORDS

- Childhood violence • Childhood trauma • Children living in war zones
- Violence and brain development

KEY POINTS

- Among world's approximately 2 billion children, estimated 1.00 to 1.25 billion experience violence annually.
- The percent of the world's children living in war zones increased by approximately 75% from 1990 (200 million) to 2016 (357 million) and continues to grow.
- Armed conflict produces changes in the architecture and neuroendocrine functioning of a child's brain, producing significant learning and behavioral disorders.
- The long-term impacts of abuse, violence, and neglect include mental, cognitive, behavioral, physical, metabolic, neurologic, and immunologic sequelae, which may manifest long after childhood.

WHAT CONSTITUTES VIOLENCE AGAINST CHILDREN AND HOW PREVALENT IS IT?

The traditional categorization of violence and its impact on child well-being has evolved, as has the conceptualization of the blueprint for peace and prosperity for people and the planet. The world's goals are articulated in the 2030 Agenda for Sustainable Development, adopted by all United Nations Member States in 2015.[1] The 17 Sustainable Development Goals, which are an urgent call for action by all countries (low income, low to medium income, medium income, and high income), encompass a global partnership. There is a recognition that, to achieve true child well-being and absence from violence against children, there needs to be a focus on the elimination of poverty and other deprivations. The strategies that must go hand in hand include those that improve health and education, decrease inequality, and spur economic growth, all while tackling global problems, such as climate change and working to

[a] Hackensack Meridian School of Medicine, 340 Kingsland Street, Nutley, NJ 07110, USA; [b] New York Academy of Medicine, 1216 Fifth Avenue, New York, NY 10029, USA; [c] New York Academy of Medicine, Mailman School of Public Health, Columbia University, SUNY Upstate Medical University, 1216 Fifth Avenue, New York, NY 10029, USA
* Corresponding author.
E-mail address: bonita.stanton@shu.edu

Pediatr Clin N Am 68 (2021) 339–349
https://doi.org/10.1016/j.pcl.2020.12.001
0031-3955/21/© 2021 Elsevier Inc. All rights reserved.

pediatric.theclinics.com

preserve our oceans and forests. The importance of using this new framework is essential to arrive at the root causes of violence and the interventions to eliminate such violence.

As discussed in the preface to this volume, the most recent World Health Organization (WHO)–Lancet Commission publication identified 5 dimensions of child rights. In this volume, we are focusing on one of these dimensions, namely, protection from violence and exploitation.[2]

The WHO estimates that approximately 53,000 children are murdered each year.[3] An estimated 1.00 to 1.25 billion children—from among the world's 2 billion children—suffer from violence each year.[4] Many overlapping definitions of violence against children exist in the literature that broadly include physical, medical, and/or psychological actions against the child and/or her or his parents or siblings, other family members, or peers.[5–9] Each of these acts of violence may be compounded by the problems inherent in poverty and the structural inequalities related to racial, ethnic, gender, religious, sexual orientation, and disability-based biases, among others. In this article we have elected to be guided by the WHO's description of the "Types of violence against children"[10]:

Most violence against children involves at least one of six main types of interpersonal violence that tend to occur at different stages in a child's development.
• Child Maltreatment (including violent punishment) involves physical, sexual and psychological/emotional violence; and neglect of infants, children and adolescents by parents, caregivers and other authority figures, most often in the home but also in settings such as schools and orphanages.
• Bullying (including cyber-bullying) is unwanted aggressive behavior by another child or group of children who are neither siblings nor in a romantic relationship with the victim. It involves repeated physical, psychological or social harm, and often takes place in schools and other settings where children gather, and online.
• Youth Violence is concentrated among children and young adults, those aged 10 to 29 years, occurs most often in community settings between acquaintances and strangers, includes bullying and physical assault with or without weapons (such as guns and knives), and may involve gang violence.
• Intimate partner violence (or domestic violence) involves physical, sexual and emotional violence by an intimate partner or ex-partner. Although males can also be victims, intimate partner violence disproportionately affects females. It commonly occurs against girls within child marriages and early/forced marriages. Among romantically involved but unmarried adolescents it is sometimes called "dating violence."
• Sexual violence includes non-consensual completed or attempted sexual contact and acts of a sexual nature not involving contact (such as voyeurism or sexual harassment); acts of sexual trafficking committed against someone who is unable to consent or refuse; and online exploitation.
• Emotional or psychological violence includes restricting a child's movements, denigration, ridicule, threats and intimidation, discrimination, rejection and other non-physical forms of hostile treatment.

Throughout this volume of *Pediatric Clinics of North America*, multiple statistics applied to some aspect of childhood violence are cited using differing timeframes, differing constituents, and different purposes. There is no correct number or percentage or timeframe because the methods for data gathering, the definitions of children, and the situations considered to be forms of child violence vary by country, author, and circumstance.[11] However, the recent Global Burden of Disease 2017[12] has used a unifying methodology to attempt to better compare data across national boundaries and yield global data (**Table 1**).

Table 1
Global prevalence, incidence, and years lived with disabilities for 2017: percentage change of age-standardized rates for 2007 to 2017

Injuries	Prevalence (Thousands) 2017 Counts	(Thousands) 2017 Counts	Years Lived with Disabilities (Thousands) 2017 Counts	Change in Age-Standardized Rates, 2007–17
Assault by firearm	2599.6 (2158.5–3151.0)	551.9 (421.7 to 725.6)	116.9 (83.8 to 159.3)	0.5% (−0.9 to 1.9)
Assault by sharp object	14,754.5 (12,033.6 to 20,359.8)	4233.0 (3265.4 to 5366.7)	475.1 (333.8 to 659.8)	−3.4% (−4.9 to −1.9)[a]
Sexual violence	238200.3 (209368.6 to 270335.5)	—	2142.0 (1447.1 to 3106.7)	0.6% (0.6 to 1.6)
Assault by other means	42,227.1 (35,479.3 to 50,750.5)	18,134.5 (15,426.3 to 21,180.0)	1827.8 (1295.0 to 2446.7)	−1.9% (−3.0 to −0.7)[a]
Conflict and terrorism	41,912.3 (28,964.3 to 59,365.8)	12,492.6 (10,797.4 to 15,087.4)	2134.0 (1438.2 to 3191.0)	−3.2% (−7.6 to 1.4)
Executions and police conflict	3680 5 (2459.9 to 5304.1)	2027.6 (1683.1 to 2486.1)	139.3 (99.1 to 197.0)	14.6% (9.9 to 31.1)[a]

[a] Percentage changes that are statistically significant.
GBD 2017 Disease and Injury Incidence and Prevalence Collaborators; Global, regional, and national incidence, prevalence, and years lived with disability for 354 diseases and injuries for 195 countries and territories, 1990-2017: a systematic analysis for the Global Burden of Disease Study 2017. Global Burden of Disease Study 2017 (GBD 2017). Global Health Metrics, 392(10159), p1826 (Table 1).

Where appropriate, we will reference this source. A national US survey of prevalence of childhood exposure to violence, crime, and abuse is instructive of the pervasiveness of this problem (**Fig. 1**). But whatever the "actual" incidence is, a substantial and unacceptable percentage of our world's children are the recipients of such treatments. In "Hidden in Plain Sight: a statistical analysis of violence against children" conducted by the United Nations International Children's Fund (UNICEF) with data from 190 nations in 2014 and what they describe as "the largest-ever compilation of data on the subject of violence against children."[13] UNICEF estimates that every year 6 among 10 children ages 2 to 14 years suffer repeated episodes of physical violence from their caregivers.[13–15] An estimated three-quarters of children ages 2 to 4 years' experience "violent discipline," for example, corporal or psychological punishment.[15] In a study conducted in the United States examining a single year, the investigators found that nearly one-half (48%) of the children had been involved in some form of violence to themselves or someone in their families.[16] An international survey found that 18% of females and 8% of boys are exposed to sexual abuse.[17] Lansford and Deater-Deckard[7] found that 63% of caregivers reported that 1 or more persons in the household had used corporal means for punishment of their children in the prior month. Moreover, the reliability of such reporting is difficult to assess because the numbers reported by government reports compared with those obtained by self-report vary considerably. For example, Stoltenborgh and associates[17,18] found that children were 75 times more likely to report physical abuse and 30 times more likely to report sexual abuse than were government reports. Given this grim reality, it is clear that addressing the rights of children will require the full participation of communities, parents, and children to understand the context of the use of corporal punishment and how to reframe, with their full participation, alternative methods of education and discipline.

ANOTHER FORM OF VIOLENCE AGAINST CHILDREN: ARMED CONFLICT

Having stated that we intend to use the WHO definition of violence of children, we are immediately making 1 exception; we are adding a seventh category of armed conflict.

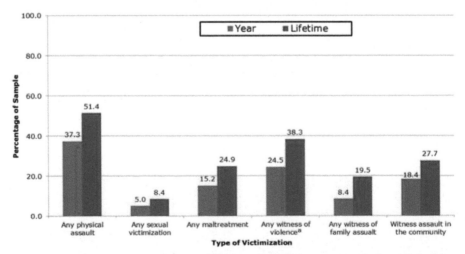

Fig. 1. Children's exposure to violence: percentage victimized 2014. [a] Excludes indirect exposure to violence. (Finkelhor, D., Turner, H. A., Shattuck, A., &. Hamby, S. L. (2015) Prevalence of childhood exposure to violence, crime, and abuse: Results from the national survey of children's exposure to violence. JAMA Pediatric, 169(8), 746 754.)

Confounding our understanding of the impact of child violence on a child's subsequent life, are the scope and magnitude of immediate, short-term and long-term sequalae of violence owing to armed conflict. Armed conflict between nations has been and remains a consistent feature of the geopolitical landscape of the twentieth and twenty-first centuries. Although the number of nations involved in armed conflicts has decreased in recent decades (i.e., from 66 countries in 1990 to 52 in 2016), the percent of the world's children living in war zones increased by about 75% during this time. In 1990, 200 million children lived in war zones, whereas in 2016 that number had increased to 357 million children[19] and to 420 million children in 2017.[20]

From 1946 to 2016, the world endured 280 armed conflicts, but much of the literature describing these conflicts did not specifically address outcomes for children and youth. Moreover, analysis of this literature is complicated by the lack of consensus defining "armed conflict".[21] Other variables must be considered that are less relevant during times of peace. For example, during armed conflicts not only might the family be forced to leave their homes to seek safety, the child may be forced to leave his or her family, traveling with another family, or even alone.[22,23] Such children are likely to be more vulnerable to infection, psychological trauma, and abuse, all the more so when economic and/or political sanctions are imposed. Likewise, children may be the victims of significant and widely variable physical injuries. If they are able to reach health care facilities, they may or may not be accompanied by a family member and the health care facility may or may not have the skills, equipment, and/or supplies needed to care for the child.[21]

Another feature of injuries occurring among children as a result of armed conflict are the types of head injuries that they endure. These injuries differ substantially from those that are encountered outside of armed conflict and, thus, appropriate treatment may not be readily available.[24] Descriptive studies of the type of injuries involving children and how they differ from those suffered by adults are relatively common, although descriptions of long-term functioning are uncommon—and even nonexistent for some injuries. Those that do exist suggest that the sequalae are more severe and cover a broader range of symptoms compared with head injuries seen among adult victims.[21,25,26] There are a limited number of long-term descriptions of the impact of chemical and/or biologic weapons. Toxic exposures not characterized as weapons may occur under conditions of war, displacement, and severe poverty and merit attention to avert the deleterious effects on children who, by virtue of their stage of development, are particularly vulnerable. A lack of access to vaccinations, prior immunity, and limited access to water and sanitation, particularly in cases of physical displacement of the child, represent additional war-related assaults on a health-promoting childhood.[21]

Land mines are a common cause of war injury for children, affecting about as many children as adults. In 1 study conducted in Afghanistan, children were found to be more likely to suffer injuries from unexploded ordinances than were adults.[27] When the mines have been planted in playgrounds, a not uncommon war tactic, children are even more likely to be the victims[21] (**Fig. 2**).

Finally, the long-term success of children is further impeded by the need for many children and youth to drop out of school during the conflict for safety, dislocation, and/or destruction of the school building. Depending on the duration of the educational lapse, some studies found lower long-term educational outcomes for these children.[28] Compounding the direct effects of the war on the health of the children, parents in active duty in some studies were more likely to abuse their children during the period of active duty and after[29,30] and their children were at an increased risk for violent behavior and weapon carrying in high school.[31] Mortality in general for children

KILLING AND MAIMING OF CHILDREN

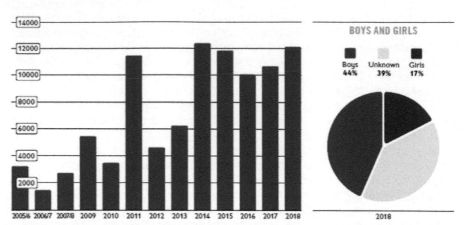

Fig. 2. The number of children killed and maimed in conflict, by year, and breakdown by sex in 2018. (Save the Children, Stop the War on Children 2020: Gender Matters. (2020) p. 20.)

increased when their country was engaged in an armed conflict, typically with a greater increase among those children greater than 5 years of age.[21,32]

Kadir and colleagues[21] summarize that armed conflict has a significant and pervasive negative impact on children and point to the literature documenting the changes in the architecture and neuroendocrine functioning in a child's brain after exposure to armed conflict. These changes are associated with changes in physiology, learning, and behavior which in turn seed maladaptive behaviors that endure through adulthood.[33] As called out by the recent *Lancet Commission on Adolescent Health and Wellbeing*,[34] adolescents may be especially vulnerable to these neurocognitive insults given the magnitude of change in neurodevelopment occurring during adolescence (and young adulthood.)

WHAT ARE THE POSSIBLE CONSEQUENCES OF VIOLENCE AGAINST CHILDREN?

The consequences of abuse, violence, and/or neglect, including developmental delays, mental health issues, delayed cognitive development, or other problems in school performance, involvement in sex trafficking and/or delinquent behavior, are legion and significant, although the child may not overtly display these outcomes for many years. All forms of child maltreatment described elsewhere in this article may be associated with mental and physical health problems for the recipient long past childhood.[4,35–41] Exposure to violence as a child is associated with an increased risk of adult chronic diseases, such as cancer, cardiovascular disease, diabetes, and chronic lung disease.[4,42] Other studies suggest that the traumatic stress inflicted on the child victim may result in impaired brain development, immune status, metabolic systems, and inflammatory responses.[43] The economic estimates of the lifetime costs associated with child physical abuse have been reported to be many billions of dollars. For example, in 1 study[44] the cost of childhood maltreatment was estimated to be $124 billion dollars in 1 year. Although historically there has been concern that questioning children and adolescents about abusive episodes in which they have been the victim may be upsetting, there is growing evidence it may be therapeutic for many.[45,46]

There is growing interest in polyvictimization, defined as more than 1 victimization episode across childhood and youth. Victimization at some point during childhood and adolescence is common. In 1 study among nearly 2000 children and youth in the United States, almost 80% reported at least 1 episode of victimization thus far in their lives, with a mean of 3.7 episodes. The authors found that both the total number of episodes of victimization and the severity of the act of victimization were associated with greater lifelong distress.[47] Despite this evidence, there is also some suggestion that, under certain circumstances, a survival advantage may result from different types of abuse. For example, some evidence exists supporting the hypothesis that children who are neglected without additional abuse may actually function more poorly than do children who are both neglected and abused. This finding should not be misinterpreted to imply that further abuse benefits the child, but rather that the severely neglected child who does not receive additional attention, even negative attention, may require additional support services, such as language development.[48]

PREVENTING VIOLENCE AGAINST CHILDREN

Although beyond the scope of this article (see other articles in the issue for an in-depth discussion of Violence Prevention), in any conversation about the consequences of violence against children, one must continuously keep in mind the overarching importance of the prevention of violence against children. Without question, responding to the child or children who have suffered violence is essential, but treatment of the child harmed by violence would not be necessary if the violence had not occurred.[49,50] In recent years, there has been considerable global emphasis on prevention of violence against children.[51–54] The WHO's Global Campaign for Violence Prevention has adopted as one of its major foci the prevention of violence again children.[55] In partnership with the International Society for the Prevention of Childhood and Neglect, the WHO coauthored "Preventing child maltreatment: a guide to taking action and generating evidence."[56] The approach is creative in that it is advocating for prevention programs while at the same time offering readers guidance as to how to collect evidence that violence against children is occurring to increase the case for support for such initiatives. In an international collaboration that published *INSPIRE: Seven strategies for ending violence against children,* the participating organizations identify specific strategies that have shown success in decreasing violence against children.[57] UNICEF is likewise deeply committed to the prevention of violence impacting children and to the intentional inclusion of the voices of children in drafting the solutions to entrenched problems such as violence using the approaches of UNICEF Child Friendly Cities.[58,59]

SUMMARY OF GLOBAL BURDEN OF VIOLENCE AND CHILDREN

An untold number of children are personally impacted by violence every year. The total percent and number of children directly impacted is staggering as are types of violent assaults that they confront. Although there are countless local, national, and international organizations concerned with violence against children, the reported numbers of children impacted is steadily growing. Some of this growth is simply because there are more children in the world and international reporting has increased. However, there is reason to believe that, whether through domestic violence, environmental violence, or armed conflict, children are as frequently victimized now as they have been in the past and there are at least some data supporting the notion that they are in fact increasingly victimized. These data are a compelling argument that we must act swiftly and globally to prevent such violence.

DISCLOSURE

The authors have nothing to disclose.

REFERENCES

1. World Health Organization. Transforming our world: the 2030 Agenda for Sustainable Development. 2015. Available at: https://sustainabledevelopment.un.org/post2015/transformingourworld. Accessed May 23, 2020.
2. Clark H, Coll-Seck AW, Banerjee A, et al. A future for the world's children: a WHO-UNICEF lancet commission. Lancet 2020;395:605–58.
3. World Health Organization. Violence and injury prevention: prevention of child maltreatment. WHO Scales up child prevention and maltreatment activities. Available at: https://www.who.int/violence_injury_prevention/violence/activities/child_maltreatment/en/. Accessed May 9, 2020.
4. Hillis SD, Mercy JA, Saul J, et al. THRIVES: a global technical package to prevent violence against children. Atlanta (GA): Centers for Disease Control and Prevention; 2015.
5. Chiang LF, Kress H, Summer SA, et al. Violence Against Children Surveys (VACS): towards a global surveillance system. Inj Prev 2016;22(Suppl 1):i17–22.
6. Bott S, Guedes a, Godwin M, et al. Violence against women in Latin America and the Caribbean: a comparative analysis of population-based data from 12 countries. Washington, DC: Pam American Health Organization; 2012.
7. Lansford JE, Deater-Deckard K. Childrearing discipline and violence in developing countries. Child Development 2012;83:62–75.
8. Krug EG, Dahlberg LI, Dahlberg JA, et al, editors. World report on violence and health. Geneva (Switzerland): World Health Organization; 2002.
9. Lozano RM, Naghavi M, Foreman K, et al. Global and regional mortality from 235 causes of death for 20 age groups in 1990 and 2010: a systematic analysis for the Global Burden of Disease Study 2010. Lancet 2012;380(9859):2095–128.
10. World Health Organization. Violence against children 2019. Available at: https://www.who.int/news-room/fact-sheets/detail/violence-against-children. Accessed May 23, 2020.
11. Jud A, Fegert JM, Finkelhor D. On the incidence and prevalence of child maltreatment: a research agenda. Child Adolesc Psychiatry Ment Health 2016;11:17.
12. Global Health Data Exchange. Global Burden of disease study 2017. Available at: http://ghdx.healthdata.org/gbd-2017. Accessed May 23, 2020.
13. United Nations Children's Fund. Hidden in plain sight: a statistical analysis of violence against children. 2014. Available at: https://data.unicef.org/resources/hidden-in-plain-sight-a-statistical-analysis-of-violence-against-children/. Accessed May 23, 2020.
14. United Nations Children 's Fund. Ending violence against children: six strategies for action. New York: UNICEF; 2014. Available at: https://www.unicef.org/publications/index_74866.html. Accessed May 23, 2020.
15. United Nations Children's Fund. A familiar face. Violence in the lives of children and adolescents. New York: UNICEF; 2017. Available at: https://www.unicef.org/publications/files/Violence_in_the_lives_of_children_and_adolescents.pdf. Accessed June 2, 2020.
16. Finkelhor D, Turner HA, Shattuck MA, et al. Violence, crime, and abuse exposure in a national sample of children and youth: an update. JAMA Pediatr 2013;167:514–21.

17. Stoltenborgh MA. Global perspective on child sexual abuse: meta-analysis of prevalence around the world. Child Maltreat 2011;16:79–101.

18. Stoltenborgh MA, Bakermans-Kranenburg MJ, van Lizendoorn MH, et al. Cultural-geographical differences in the occurrence of child physical abuse? A meta-analysis of global prevalence. Int J Psychol 2013;48:81–94.

19. Gray A. World Economic Forum. What you need to know about the world's youth, in 7 charts. 2018. Available at: https://Weforum.org/agenda/2018/what-you-need-to-know-about-the-worlds-young-people-in-7-charts/. Accessed June 2, 2020.

20. Lu J. The number of children affected by conflict is Skyrocketing UN DISPATCH United nations news & Commentary global news Forum 2019. Available at: https://www.undispatch.com/children-affected-by-conflict/. Accessed June 2, 2020.

21. Kadir A, Shenoda S, Goldhagen J. Effects of armed conflict on child health and development: a systematic review. PLoS One 2019;14(1). https://doi.org/10.1371/journal.pone.0210071. Accessed June 2, 2020.

22. Marquard L, Kramor A, Fischer F, et al. Health status and disease burden of unaccompanied asylum seeking adolescence in Bielefeld, Germany: cross-sectional pilot study. Trop Med Int Health 2016–;21(2):210–8. PMID 26610271. Available at: https://doi.org/10.1111/cch. Accessed June 2, 2020.

23. ISSOP Migration Working Group. ISSOP position statement on migrant child health. Child Care Health Dev 2018–;44(1):161–70. PMID 28736840. Available at: https://doi.org/10.1111/cch. Accessed June 2, 2020.

24. Woods K, Russell RJ, Bree S, et al. The pattern of pediatric trauma on operations. JR Army Med Corps 2012;158(1):34–7.

25. Momeni AZ, Aminjavaheri M. Skin manifestations of mustard gas in a group of 14 children and teenagers; a clinical study. Int J Dermatol 1994;33(3):184–7.

26. Guha Sapir D, Rodriguez-Lianos JM, Hicks MH, et al. Civilian deaths from weapons used in the Syrian conflict. BMI 2015;351:h4736.

27. Bilukha OO, Brennan M, Woodruff BA. Death and injury from landmines and unexploded ordinance in Afghanistan. JAMA 2003;290;650–3.

28. Rodriguez C, Sanchez F. Armed conflict exposure. human capital investments. and child labor: evidence from Columbia. Deference Peace Econ 2012;23(2): 161–84.

29. Rabenhorst MM, McCarthy RJ, Thomsen CJ, et al. Child maltreatment among U.S. air force parents deployed in support of operation Iraq Freedom Operation Enduring Freedom. Child Maltreat 2015;201(1):61–71. Available at: https://pubmed.ncbi.nlm.nih.gov/25424846/. Accessed May 23, 2020.

30. Rentz ED, Marshall SW, Loomis D, et al. Effect of deployment on the occurrence of child maltreatment in military and nonmilitary families. Am J Epidemiol 2007–; 165(10):1199–206. PMID173297716. Available at: https://doi.org/10.1093/aje/kwm008. Accessed June 2, 2020.

31. Sullivan K, Oapp G, Gitreath TD, et al. Substance abuse and other adverse outcomes for military-connected youth in California: results from a large-scale normative population survey. JAMA Pediatr 2015;169(10):922–8. Available at: https://pubmed.ncbi.nlm.nih.gov/26280338/. Accessed June 2, 2020.

32. Guha-Sapir D, van Panhuis WG. Conflict-related mortality: an analysis of 37 datasets. Disasters 2004;28(4):18–28. Available at: https://onlinelibrary.wiley.com/doi/abs/10.1111/j.0361-3666.2004.00267.x. Accessed June 2, 2020.

33. Shonkoff JP, Garner AS, Siegel NS, et al. The lifelong effects of early childhood adversity and toxic stress. Pediatrics 2012;129(1):e232–46. PMID 22201156.

34. Patton GC, Sawyer SM, Santelli JS, et al. Our future: a Lancet commission on adolescent health and wellbeing. Lancet 2016;385(10036):2423–78.
35. Hillberg T, Hamilton-Giachritsis C, Dixon L. Review of meta-analysis on the association between child sexual abuse and adult mental health difficulties: a systematic approach. Trauma Violence Abuse 2011;12:38–49.
36. Kaplan SJ, Pelcovitz D, Labruna V. Child and adolescent abuse and neglect research; a review of the past 10 years. Part 1: physical and emotional abuse and neglect. J Am Acad Child Adolesc Psychiatr 1999;38:1214–22.
37. Roemmele M, Messman-Moore TL. Child abuse, early maladaptive schemes, and risky sexual behavior in college women. J Child Sex Abus 2011;20:264–83.
38. Lalor K, McElvaney R. Child sexual abuse, links to later sexual exploitation/high-risk sexual behavior, and prevention/treatment programs. Trauma Violence Abus 2010;11:159–77.
39. Senn TE, Carey MP. Child maltreatment and women's adult sexual risk behavior: childhood sexual abuse as a unique risk factor. Child Maltreat 2010;15:324–35.
40. Wilson HW, Widom CS. An examination of risky sexual behavior and HIV in victims of child abuse and neglect: a 30-year follow-up. Health Psychol 2008;27: 149–58.
41. Nelson EC, Heath AC, Madden PAF, et al. Association between self-reported childhood sexual abuse and adverse psychosocial outcomes: results from a twin study. Arch Gen Psychiatry 2002;59:139–45.
42. Krug EG, Dahlberg LL, Mercy JA, et al, editors. World report on violence and health. Geneva (Switzerland): World Health Organization;2002.
43. Anda RF, Butchart A, Felitti VJ, et al. Building a framework for global surveillance of the public health implications of adverse childhood experiences. Am J Prev Med 2010;39(1):93–8.
44. Fang X, Brown DS, Florence CS, et al. The economic burden of child maltreatment in the United States and implications for prevention. Child Abuse Negl 2012;36:156–65.
45. Finkelhor D, Vanderminden J, Turner H, et al. Upset among youth in response to questions about exposure to violence, sexual assault and family maltreatment. Child Abuse Negl 2014;38:217–23.
46. Graham-Bermann SA, Kulkarni MR, Kanukolu SN. Is disclosure therapeutic for children following exposure to traumatic violence? J Interpers Violence 2011; 26(5):1056–76.
47. Finkelhor D, Ormrod RK, Turner HA. Lifetime assessment of poly-victimization in a national sample of children and youth. Child Abuse Negl 2009;33(74):403–11.
48. O'Hara M, Lori Legano L, Homel P, et al. Children neglected: where cumulative risk theory fails. Child Abuse Negl 2015;45:1–8.
49. Fluke JD, Goldman PS, Shriberg J, et al. Systems, strategies, and interventions for sustainable long-term care and protection of children with a history of living outside of family care. Child Abuse Negl 2012;36(10):722–31.
50. Centers for Disease Control and Prevention. Essentials for childhood: steps to create safe, stable, nurturing relationships and environments. Atlanta, GA: Centers for Disease Control and Prevention; 2014. Available at: https://www.cdc.gov/violenceprevention/childabuseandneglect/essentials.html. Accessed May 24, 2020.
51. CARE, Save the Children, and the Consultative Group on Early Childhood Care and Development. 2012. "The essential package: holistically addressing the needs of young vulnerable children and their caregivers affected by HIV/AIDS."

52. Mercy JA, Hills S, Butchart A, et al. "Interpersonal violence: global impact and paths to prevention" (Chapter 5). In: Mock CN, Nugent R, Kobusingye O, et al, editors. Injury Prevention and Environmental Health, 3rd edition. Disease control priorities, vol. 7. Washington, DC: The International Bank for Reconstruction and Development/The World Bank; 2017.

53. World Health Organization. Milestones of a global Campaign for violence prevention 2002. Available at: https://www.who.int/violence_injury_prevention/publications/violence/publication_milestones/en/. Accessed May 22, 2020.

54. United Nations Children's Fund. Ending violence against children: six strategies for action. September 2014. New York: UNICEF; 2014.

55. World Health Organization. 8th Milestones of a Global Campaign for Violence Prevention. Ottawa, Canada, 19-20 October 2017. Available at: https://www.who.int/violence_injury_prevention/violence/8th_milestones_meeting/en/. Accessed May 23, 2020.

56. World Health Organization and International Society for Prevention of Childhood Abuse and Neglect. Preventing child maltreatment: a guide to taking action and generating evidence 2006. Available at: https://www.who.int/violence_injury_prevention/publications/violence/child_maltreatment/en/. Accessed May 23, 2020.

57. World Health Organization and the Pan American Health Organization. INSPIRE: seven strategies for ending violence against children. Geneva (Switzerland): WHO; 2016. Available at: https://www.who.int/publications-detail/inspire-seven-strategies-for-ending-violence-against-children. Accessed May 23, 2020.

58. United Nations Children's Fund. Preventing and responding to violence against children and adolescents: theory of change 2017. Available at: https://www.unicef.org/protection/files/UNICEF_VAC_ToC_2_pager_WEB_051217.pdf. Accessed May 23, 2020.

59. United Nations Children's Fund. Child Friendly Cities Initiative. Available at: https://childfriendlycities.org/. Accessed May 24, 2020.

Operating Principles and Competencies for Engagement in Global/Local Settings

Danielle Laraque-Arena, MD[a,b,c,d],*

KEYWORDS

- Faculty competencies • Operating principles • Global health
- Implementation research

KEY POINTS

- Operating principles and faculty competencies should guide global and local educational, research, clinical, and administrative endeavors with local and global partners.
- Faculty competencies for those engaging in global/local efforts should adhere to guidance on values/ethics, roles/responsibilities, communication, team building, and teamwork, with attention to special considerations.
- Five operating principles include population specifics, political/social context that may polarize efforts, applying positive strategies, persistence, and partnerships in achieving improved health status for populations.

The discussion of *Ending The War Against Children: The Rights Of Children To Live Free of Violence* is grounded in operating principles guiding the framework for actions on behalf of children as well as the competencies that health care professionals should possess in order to skillfully and ethically address the needs of children affected by war and violence. First published in 2011,[1] and used as the basis for the book *Principles of Global Child Health: Education and Research*,[2] 5 operating principles are described for health professionals engaged in clinical, educational, research, or administrative global/local efforts involving the health of children, their families, and communities.

The 5 operating principles attempt to set the context for analysis and interventions addressing key avoidable morbidity and mortality realities and guide the application of tangible steps for the reduction of poor health outcomes in all populations. In the case of the current focus on violence against children, readers are urged to examine the

[a] New York Academy of Medicine, New York, NY, USA; [b] Mailman School of Public Health, Columbia University, New York, NY, USA; [c] Injury Free Coalition for Kids, National Program, New York, NY, USA; [d] SUNY Upstate Medical University, Syracuse, NY, USA
* 1216 Fifth Avenue, New York, NY 10029.
E-mail addresses: Dlaraque-arena@nyam.org; dl3365@cumc.columbia.edu

Pediatr Clin N Am 68 (2021) 351–356
https://doi.org/10.1016/j.pcl.2020.12.002
0031-3955/21/© 2020 Elsevier Inc. All rights reserved.
pediatric.theclinics.com

case studies presented within the framework of the overriding principles of engagement and the competencies of the stakeholders in order to draw organizational learnings from these described experiences.

These operating principles, or 5 Ps, find support in the published literature and are as listed as follows:

1. The importance of population-specific, local data that support a baseline analysis of the problem being addressed with the disaggregation of data on a variety of demographics and characteristics to yield population-specific and culturally-specific approaches and evaluations of intended outcomes[3-7]
2. The need to address the concept of polarization, which refers to opposing forces that create seemingly antagonistic positions, but must be understood to yield the identification of obstacles and threats to improved outcomes[1,8]
3. The need for positive strategies that allow the bar to be set high for proactive, preventative, and strength-based approaches to solving entrenched problems and, in doing so, being intentionally inclusive of voices previously excluded[9]
4. Persistence, a necessary component of efforts aimed at eliminating historical and current injustices linked to poor health outcomes, fueled by data that continuously monitor and illuminate progress[10]
5. Finally, the fifth component of achieving improved health outcomes is the necessity of partnerships that are genuine, respectful, culturally relevant, legal, and ethical and help drive sustainable change and define principled planning that is bi/multidirectional.[11-15]

This article proposes these principles as guidelines for evaluating the authenticity of engagement with individuals, communities, universities, governmental agencies, nongovernmental agencies, and the array of stakeholders addressing child health and child rights.[16]

The operating principles ideally are paired with distinct competencies of faculty in educational, research, and clinical settings. The premise for the operating principles and the need for well-defined competencies is that healthy children are the anchor for sustainable development.[17,18] In order to achieve the outcomes of child health and well-being, research, clinical care, educational foundation, and administrative oversight must be taught and measured by articulated competencies. These competencies are described in other publications[18] and are summarized here.

Five areas identify and define 4 distinct faculty competencies. These competencies are in the realm of global administrative, education, research, and clinical spheres and invoke actions to be taken. Developed initially by the Academic Pediatric Association Global Health Task Force and endorsed by the American Academy of Pediatrics, each of the targeted areas of competency addresses values/ethics, roles/responsibilities, communication, team building and teamwork, and special considerations, as described[18-22]:

- The values and ethics defined in each of the competencies relate to a shared purpose, committed to safe, efficient, and effective systems of care, education, and research.[18] Salient points in this domain are the need to align the goals and objectives of all partners/stakeholders (eg, host country and community) and, in doing so, assure bi/multidirectional relationships that do not shift the power differential away from the country/partner that may be perceived as having fewer resources. A reliance on addressing social determinants of health is a key tenet, with the inclusion of a multitude of voices with a stake in the outcome of the endeavor, respecting cultural and ethical contexts.

- The next competency is the requirement that faculty be explicit regarding their roles and responsibilities, recognizing the limits of one's professional expertise, which allows for respectful partnerships in support of coordination and cooperation of efforts to improve health status. Cultural humility in this context is critical, understanding that all participants have something to learn from each other. Cultural arrogance, for example, in presuming that 1 party is all knowing, must be managed, allowing for openness to innovation, creativity, and culturally relevant approaches to education, research, clinical care, and the distribution of power in administrative functions. Equally important is the clear articulation of the expected results from each of the parties. The conceptual framework of implementation research is particularly relevant in this regard and relates to the responsibilities of each party and is likely a precondition to obtaining the desired changes in outcomes (clinical, service, research, advocacy, and policy). Three possible outcome buckets have been described by Proctor and colleagues[23]: implementation outcomes, service outcomes, and client/clinical outcomes (**Fig. 1**).
  - According to Proctor and colleagues, the definition of *implementation outcomes* is "the effects of deliberate and purposive actions to implement the new treatments, practices, and services." The function of such research is to indicate the success of the research, the proximal indicators of the implementation processes, and the intermediate outcomes with regard to the service system or clinical outcomes in effectiveness and quality of care research. In the implementation outcomes bucket are included the indicators of acceptability, adoption, appropriateness, costs, feasibility, fidelity, penetration, and sustainability. These concepts are important in framing the trust proposition because they go to the heart of what most communities and patients/clients seek, that is, caring about whether or not a treatment, a research finding, a teaching methodology can be translated into practice to positively influence the outcomes at the population level for maximum impact.
  - Service outcomes are those defined by the Institute of Medicine[24] as 6 quality improvement aims and describe the extent to which a service is safe, effective, patient-centered, timely, efficient, and equitable. Within the roles and

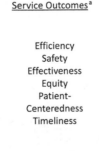

Implementation Outcomes	Service Outcomes[a]	Client/Patient Outcome
Acceptability	Efficiency	Satisfaction
Adoption	Safety	Function
Appropriateness	Effectiveness	Symptomatology
Costs	Equity	
Feasibility	Patient-Centeredness	
Fidelity	Timeliness	
Penetration		
Sustainability		

Fig. 1. Types of outcomes in implementation research. [a]Institute of Medicine Standards of Care. (*Adapted from* Proctor, 2011.)

responsibilities component of the defined competencies, adherence to the service outcomes is important.
- ○ The client/patient outcomes relate to satisfaction, function, and symptomatology. Attentiveness to these outcomes is a component of the roles/responsibilities of educators, researchers, clinicians, and administrators.
- A third competency, faculty/researcher/educator/clinician commitment to frank, transparent, and open communication to improve organizational functioning and interactions among the various disciplines and sectors, is deemed essential. The value of effective communication is replete in the literature.[25–27] Emphasis on establishing bi/multidirectional communication in addressing the global problem of violence against children is evident in understanding the local context of such violence, its root causes, and the possible community-based solutions and youth-driven solutions as exemplified by models, such as the Child Friendly Cities Initiative of UNICEF USA.[28] Mentorship, teaching, and learning should engage active listening in addressing difficult and emotionally taxing discussions, such as child marriage, classism, racism, and sexism, The rendering of concrete, locally valuable output, such as reports, policies, research papers, curricula, and other educational materials supports effective communication in community and global contexts and is supportive of the process of building trust.
- Faculty valuing teamwork that improves the effectiveness of any academic endeavor is critical to effectively address complex problems, such as violence and war against children. In the twenty-first century, the term, *team science*, has become common. This term denotes "cross-disciplinary engagement and collaboration and the longer-term interaction of groups of investigators."[29,30] The science aspect is concerned with improving understanding of the effectiveness of collaborative efforts and its application to the analysis of research, training, and community-based initiatives to render societal needs. The praxis of team science is understanding the experience of leading, training, and engaging in diverse situations and settings (eg, global health settings) in tackling a particular clinical or public health problem. Readers of this issue on violence against children as demonstrated by case studies are urged to view these presentations within the lens of team effectiveness and the lessons learned from navigating the complexities of the circumstances faced by children and teens.
- Finally, there is a need to understand and prepare for context and complex special considerations. The United Nations (UN) has defined complex humanitarian emergency as "a humanitarian crisis in a country, region, or society where there is total or considerable breakdown of authority resulting from internal or external conflict and which requires an international response that goes beyond the mandate or capacity of any single and/or ongoing UN country program."[31] These circumstances are determined by the political situation, cultural milieu, and resource setting. The organization, Médecins Sans Frontières, the winner of the Nobel Peace Prize, Indira Gandhi Prize, and Lasker-Bloomberg Public Service Award, has mastered special considerations with adherence to the operating principles and professional competence elements discussed in this article.[32]

This article does not seek to detail the application of the subcomponents of professional competencies specific to administrative, clinical, research, and educational medical faculty roles; these are described elsewhere.[2,18–22] The article sets in motion the framework by which these competencies should be viewed and applied. Readers of this issue are encouraged to analyze and read the specific articles and the lessons derived, keeping the operating principles and competencies in mind.

CLINICS CARE POINTS

- In caring for children and families, clinicians who apply the operating principles and display the faculty competencies described are likely to engender patient satisfaction with care.
- While the relationship between patient satisfaction and quality of care is complex, patient satisfaction is recognized as an important component of care.

DISCLOSURE

The author has nothing to disclose.

REFERENCES

1. Laraque D. Global child health: reaching the tipping point for all children. Acad Pediatr 2011;11:226–33.
2. Laraque-Arena D, Stanton B, editors. Principles of global child health: education and research. Itasca (IL): Publisher, American Academy of Pediatrics; 2019.
3. GBD 2017: a fragile world. Lancet 2018;392(10159):1683–2138.
4. Patton GC, Sawyer SM, Santelli JS, et al. Our Future: A Lancet commission on adolescent health and wellbeing. Lancet 2016;387:2423–78.
5. Patel V, Saxena S, Lund C, et al. The Lancet Commission on global mental health and sustainable development. Lancet 2018;392(10157):1553–98.
6. Goldhagen J, Remo R, Bryant T, et al. The health status of southern children: a neglected regional disparity. Pediatrics 2005;116:e746–53.
7. McCord C, Freeman HP. Excess mortality in Harlem. N Engl J Med 1990;322:173–7.
8. Thompson FJ. Health reform, polarization, and public administration. Public Adm Rev 2013;73(S1):S3–12.
9. Knitzer J. Advocacy and the children's crisis. Am J Orthop 1971;41(5):799–806.
10. Knitzer J. Child advocacy: a perspective. Am J Orthopsychiatry 1976;46(2):200–16.
11. Laraque D, Barlow B, Durkin M, et al. Injury prevention in an urban setting: challenges and successes. Bull N Y Acad Med 1995;72:16–30.
12. Laraque D, Barlow B, Davidson L, et al. The Central Harlem playground injury prevention project: a model for change. Am J Public Health 1994;84:1691–2.
13. Laraque D, Barlow B, Durkin M, et al. Children who are shot: a 30-year experience. J Pediatr Surg 1995;30:1072–5 [Discussion: 1075–6].
14. Pressley JC, Barlow B, Durkin M, et al. A national program for injury prevention in children and adolescents: the injury free coalition for kids. J Urban Health 2005;82:389–402.
15. Available at: https://www.gavi.org/our-alliance/operating-model/gavis-partnership-model; Accessed August 2, 2020.
16. United Nations, Convention on the Rights of the Child. Available at: https://www.ohchr.org/en/professionalinterest/pages/crc.aspx. Accessed August 2, 2020.
17. Statement of endorsement, faculty competencies for global health. Pediatrics 2015;135:E1535. Available at: https://pediatrics.aappublications.org/content/135/6/e1535/tab-e-letters.
18. Preface: domains of competency in global health. In: Laraque-Arena D, Stanton B, editors. Principles of global child health: education and research. American Academy of Pediatrics; 2019. p. 97–101.

19. O'Callahan C. Global health administrative competencies. In: Laraque-Arena D, Stanton B, editors. Principles of global child health: education and research. American Academy of Pediatrics; 2019. p. 103–13.
20. Kurbasic MP. Global health education competencies. In: Laraque-Arena D, Stanton B, editors. Principles of global child health: education and research. American Academy of Pediatrics; 2019. p. 115–9.
21. Etzel RA. Global health research competencies. In: Laraque-Arena D, Stanton B, editors. Principles of global child health: education and research. American Academy of Pediatrics; 2019. p. 121–32.
22. Domachowske JB, Stewart-Ibarra AM, Domachowske ET, et al. Global health clinical competencies. In: Laraque-Arena D, Stanton B, editors. Principles of global child health: education and research. American Academy of Pediatrics; 2019. p. 133–56.
23. Proctor E, Silmere H, Raghavan R, et al. Outcomes for implementation research: conceptual distinctions, measurement challenges, and research agenda. Adm Policy Ment Health 2011;38:65–76.
24. Institute of Medicine Committee on Crossing the Quality Chasm. Crossing the quality chasm: a new health system for the 21st century. Washington, DC: Institute of Medicine, National Academy Press; 2001.
25. Lingard L, Haber RJ. Teaching and learning communication in medicine: a rhetorical approach. Acad Med 1999;74(5):507–10.
26. Lobas JG. Leadership in academic medicine: capabilities and conditions for organizational success. Am J Med 2006;119(7):617–21.
27. Wahabi H, Zakaria N. Building Capacity of evidenced-based public health pravctice in king saud university: perceived challenges and opportunities. J Public Health Manag Pract 2020;26(5):428–33. Available at: www.jphmp.com.
28. Available at: https://childfriendlycities.org/. Accessed August 3, 2020.
29. Falk-Krzesinski HJ, Borner K, Contractor N, et al. Advancing the science of team science. Clin Transl Sci 2010;3(5):263–6. Available at: www.CTSJournal.com. Accessed August 3, 2020.
30. Bennett LM, Gadlin H, Levine-Finely S. NIH. August 2010. A collaboration and team science: a field guide. Available at: http://teamscience.nih.gov. Accessed August 2, 2020.
31. Burkle FM. Complex humanitarian emergencies: A review of epidemiological and response models. J Postgrad Med 2006;52:110–5.
32. Brown V, Guerin PJ, Legros D, et al. Research in complex humanitarian emergencies: the medecins sans frontieres/epicentre experience. PLoS Med 2008;5(4): e89. Available at: www.plosmedicine.org.

Violence Against Children
Recognition, Rights, Responses

Charles Oberg, MD[a], Rita Nathawad, MD[b], Shanti Raman, PhD[c],
Jeffrey Goldhagen, MD[d],*

KEYWORDS

- UN Convention on the Rights of the Child (CRC) • Violence against children (VAC)
- Child rights–based approach (CRBA) • Socioecological model and taxonomy

KEY POINTS

- Adoption of a new child rights–based approach to violence against children.
- Expansion of the sociologic model of child development to include a transsocietal sphere to address emerging global threats to child health and well-being.
- Confronting violence against children at the clinical, systems, and policy level.

INTRODUCTION

Violence against children (VAC) in all its forms is a violation of children's rights and an enormous child health issue. It has traditionally been framed in terms of abuse, neglect, maltreatment, and domestic violence—construed in the context of personal violence. However, over the past decade it has become clear that the historical construct of child abuse and neglect (CAN) is no longer fully applicable to the broad range of global assaults on children and childhood. Instead of CAN, VAC is a framework to better understand these issues and conceptualize our response—informed by the principles, standards, and norms of child rights and the UN Convention on the Rights of the Child (CRC).

As awareness of the scope of VAC increases, so too has our knowledge of its impact on child health and well-being. Evidence over the past 30 years—from neuroscience, developmental psychology, social sciences, and epidemiology—shows that VAC contributes to social, emotional, and cognitive impairments and high-risk behaviors leading to disease, disability, social problems, and premature mortality—with short-, medium-, and long-term and intergenerational consequences.[1]

[a] Global Pediatric Program, University of Minnesota, Minneapolis, MN, USA; [b] Department of Pediatrics, University of Florida, Jacksonville, FL, USA; [c] School of Women's and Children's Health, UNSW Sydney, Australia; [d] Department of Pediatrics, Division of Community and Societal Pediatrics, University of Florida, 841 Prudential Drive, Suite 900, Jacksonville, FL 32207, USA
* Corresponding author.
E-mail address: jeffrey.goldhagen@jax.ufl.edu

Pediatr Clin N Am 68 (2021) 357–369
https://doi.org/10.1016/j.pcl.2020.12.008
0031-3955/21/© 2020 Elsevier Inc. All rights reserved.

DEFINITION: A RIGHTS-BASED APPROACH TO VIOLENCE AGAINST CHILDREN

The evolution of a rights-based approach to VAC is grounded in United Nations' documents and conventions.

- The World Health Organization in1996 defined violence as the "intentional use of physical force or power, threatened or actual, against oneself, another person, or against a group or community that either results in or has a high likelihood of resulting in injury, death, psychological harm, maldevelopment or deprivation."[2]
- The 1989 UN Convention on the Rights of the Child's Article 19 defines "violence" as "all forms of physical or mental violence, injury or abuse, neglect or negligent treatment, maltreatment or exploitation, including sexual abuse."[3] The same terminology is used in the 2006 United Nations study on VAC.[4]
- The 2011 General Comment 13 to the CRC acknowledges that "the extent and intensity of violence exerted on children is alarming," and calls for "massively strengthened and expanded" efforts to "effectively put an end to these practices."
- The elimination of VAC is also called for in the 2030 Agenda for Sustainable Development, most explicitly in Target 16.2: "end abuse, exploitation, trafficking and all forms of violence against and torture of children."[5]

However, the definition of violence in these documents no longer adequately addresses the expanding scope of VAC. They fail to consider the root-cause determinants of VAC, including institutional racism, economic policies, discrimination based on sex and gender identity, poverty, globalization, climate change etc.—that so profoundly affect the survival of children and their life-course trajectory. A child rights–based definition of VAC is required to expand the perimeter of our approach to understanding and mitigating the impact of all forms of VAC. We propose, "Any intentional or unintentional action, system, or policy that violates a child's or population of children's right(s) to optimal survival and development," to begin the dialogue and discussion.

As stated in the CRC-General Comment 13, the evolution to a child rights–based approach (CRBA) to VAC "requires a shift toward respecting and promoting the human dignity and the physical and psychological integrity of children as rights-bearing individuals, rather than perceiving them primarily as victims."[6] Grounding a definition of VAC on the tenets of child rights allows for the translation of the principles and norms of human rights, social justice, and equity into practice[7]—in the domains of programs, systems, and public policies.

BACKGROUND: CHILDREN'S RIGHTS AND PROTECTION FROM VIOLENCE

On November 20, 1989, the UN General Assembly adopted the *UN Convention on the Rights of the Child*. The CRC establishes the responsibility of governments, institutions, citizens, and families, as duty-bearers, to ensure the rights of children are respected and all actions are taken to achieve the "best interest of the child" (CRC, Article 3). The CRC is the first legally binding international document to recognize the civil, political, economic, social, and cultural rights of the child. No rights articulated in the CRC take precedence—they are interdependent and indivisible. Thus, to fulfill one right requires attention to all related rights. The CRC can be categorized into 3 domains of rights: protection, promotion, and participation (**Fig. 1**).

When considering VAC, protection rights ensure children are free from all forms of violence. However, as all rights are *indivisible* and *interdependent*, promotion and participation rights are also necessary to ensure children are free from VAC. Promotion rights relate to the basic rights to life, survival, and the development of a child's full

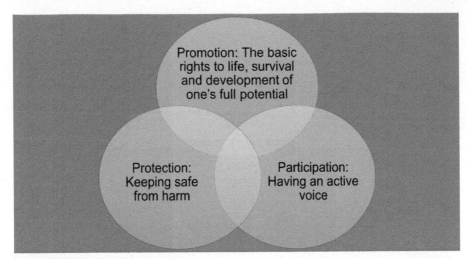

Fig. 1. Categories of children's rights.

potential. Participation rights ensure that all children have an active voice in matters that affect them. To advance a comprehensive CRBA to VAC, all rights articulated in the CRC must be fulfilled, and practices, systems, and polices must protect and promote children's rights and give voice to their stories.

DISCUSSION: CHILD RIGHTS AND VIOLENCE—A "REVISED" SOCIOECOLOGICAL TAXONOMY

The socioecological model is often used to illustrate how the lives of children and their environment interact to influence their growth and development. Children live and thrive in multiple environments, also known as ecological systems. Violence can permeate each ecological system in the form of interpersonal (child maltreatment [CM], domestic violence), community (corporal punishment, bullying, firearm injury), and societal violence (child labor, trafficking, institutionalization).[8] However, the model fails to adequately address global *transsocietal* forms of VAC that profoundly affect their optimal survival and development. Armed conflict, migration, globalization, and climate change are examples of rapidly evolving root-cause determinants of transsocietal forms of VAC that must also be addressed.[9]

Fig. 2 illustrates a revised socioecological model that provides a framework to better understand and mitigate VAC. (see **Fig. 2**).

Table 1 provides a taxonomy of VAC corresponding to children's rights with examples for each form of VAC presented.

Interpersonal Violence

Child maltreatment and domestic violence

CM, first described by Henry Kempe in the 1960s as the "Battered Child Syndrome," is the most recognized type of VAC worldwide.[10] The definition of CM includes physical abuse, sexual abuse, neglect, and emotional abuse. CM often occurs in combinations[11] and is referred to as "re-victimization" when children are exposed to repeated multiple forms of maltreatment.[12] Children with disabilities are especially at-risk.[13]

The term "domestic violence" is used to refer to intimate partner violence (IPV) but can also encompass other forms of violence including elder abuse or abuse by any

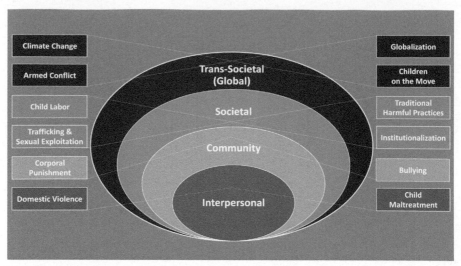

Fig. 2. Revised sociologic model for violence against children.

member of a household. Children's exposure to IPV is now recognized as a type of CM with adverse outcomes similar to other types of maltreatment.[14] Children can be both victims and witnesses to abuse.[15] In both situations, impacts are detrimental to the child's development and can affect their ability to form trusting bonds later in life.

Child rights
- CRC, Article 19, Part 1 protects children from all forms of CM using all appropriate legislative, administrative, social, and educational measures.
- CRC, Article 19, Part 2 requires measures be implemented to assure protection and includes programs to support the child and to identify, report, refer, investigate, treat, and follow-up all instances of VAC.

Community Violence

Corporal punishment
There has been significant progress toward universal prohibition of corporal punishment. Children exposed to corporal punishment experience detrimental effects, including poor academic performance, low class participation, school dropout, and declining psychosocial well-being.[16] More than 125 nations have prohibited corporal punishment in schools, and 50 countries now prohibit all corporal punishment of children.[17] Despite prohibition, corporal punishment remains highly prevalent. For example, greater than 50% of 8-year-old children in Peru and Vietnam, 75% in Ethiopia, and 90% in India reported teacher administered corporal punishment in the previous week.[18]

Child rights
- Article 43 of the CRC established The Committee on the Rights of the Child. In 2011, the Committee adopted General Comments No. 13 urged that violent and humiliating punishment of children needs to be taken seriously and addressed.[19]

Bullying
Children may face physical and emotional maltreatment from both fellow students and teachers. Bullying is repeated aggression via physical, verbal, relational, or cyber

Table 1
Taxonomy of children's rights and violence against children

Socioecological Sphere	Category of VAC	Child Rights Provisions
Interpersonal	Child maltreatment & domestic violence	CRC, Article 19—Protection from Abuse & Neglect
Community	Corporal punishment	Committee on Rights of the Child, General Comment No. 13
	Bullying	CRC, Article 29—Aims of Education
	Firearms	CRC, Article 19—Protection from Injury
Societal	Child labor	CRC, Article 32—Child Labor
	Trafficking and sexual exploitation	CRC, Article 34—Sexual Exploitation CRC, Article 35—Sale, Trafficking, & Abduction CRC Optional Protocol—Sale of Children
	Institutionalization	CRC, Article 20—Care of Children Deprived of Family Care CRC Article 37—Care in Juvenile Justice System
	Traditional harmful practices based on culture, religion, or superstition	UN General Assembly Resolution 1994/30 UN Special Representative of Secretary-General 2006 VAC Study
Trans-Societal	Armed conflict	CRC, Article 38—Armed Conflict CRC Optional Protocol—Children in Armed Conflict Geneva Convention
	Children on the move	CRC, Article 22-Refugee Children Protection & Assistance
	Globalization	Proposed establishment of New UN Commission
	Climate change	CRC, Article 6—Right to Life CRC, Article 24—Right to a Safe Environment

forms in which the targets cannot defend themselves.[20] Globally, more than 1 in 3 teenagers are regularly bullied. In some countries such as Latvia and Romania, nearly 60% admit to bullying others.[21] Technology has given rise to "cyber-bullying," a limitless platform for abuse.

Child rights
- CRC, Article 29, on the aims of education, implies that we educate children to develop attitudes and behaviors to minimize the harassment and bullying of others.[22]

Firearm-related injury and death
Firearms account for greater than 100,000 injuries and nearly 40,000 deaths annually in the United States.[23] In the United States, middle and high school–aged children are more likely to die as a result of a firearm injury than from any other single cause of death.[24] Compared with other high-income countries, American children aged 5 to 14 years are 21 times more likely to be killed by guns, and American adolescents and young adults aged 15 to 24 years are 23 times more likely to be killed by guns.[25]

Children's rights

- CRC, Article 19, Part 1 protects children from all forms of violence and injury.

Societal Violence

Child labor

Child labor is ubiquitous globally and is underpinned by poverty and deprivation of education. More than 168 million children work, with more than half of them doing hazardous tasks. Almost 10% of children in Asia and the Pacific and 21% of children in Sub-Saharan Africa are engaged in child labor.[26]

Child rights

- CRC, Article 32, Part 1 outlines the child's right against inappropriate work. States must protect children from economic exploitation that interfere with their education and/or is harmful to their physical, spiritual, or moral well-being.
- Part 2 includes provisions that regulates the conditions of employment and sanctions to ensure effective enforcement.

Trafficking and sexual exploitation

Estimates suggest that 50% of trafficked victims worldwide are children. Exploitive practices involving children include labor, domestic work, sexual exploitation, military conscription, marriage, illicit adoption, begging, and organ harvesting.[27]

Child rights

- CRC, Article 34 advocates for the protection of children from sexual exploitation. In addition, the Optional Protocol forbidding the Sale of Children, Child Prostitution and Child Pornography was added in 2000.[28]
- CRC, Article 35 encourages all nations to prevent abduction, sale, or trafficking in children.

Institutionalized children

Tens of millions of children in the world live in institutional care.[29] These children are more likely to experience violence than those living in family-based care.[30] Incarcerated youth are at even greater risk, in particular children exposed to solitary confinement,[31] and children with disabilities are at the greatest risk of abuse in institutional care.[32]

Child rights

- CRC, Article 20 provides for the special protection of a child deprived of a family environment.
- CRC, Article 23 addresses the right of "disabled" children to special care, education, and training to ensure a life lived with dignity, self-reliance, and social integration.
- CRC, Article 37 protects the rights of children detained in juvenile justice systems to be free from torture and the deprivation of liberty.

Culture and Religion

Violations of children's rights include those that are based on tradition, culture, religion, or superstition—termed "harmful traditional practices (HTP)."[33] These in particular affect the rights of women and girls, LGBTQ, and gender nonconforming individuals. The international NGO, Council on Violence against Children, recently released a report on HTP that includes examples of acid attacks, breast flattening, forced child marriage, dowry, female genital mutilation, and honor killing.[34] These harmful practices are based on long upheld patriarchal social values that act as a root cause of discrimination and violence against girls.[35]

Child rights

- UN General Assembly passed resolution 1994/30 adopting the Plan for the Elimination of Traditional Practices Affecting the Health of Women and Children.
- In 2009, UN Secretary General–appointed Special Representative on Violence Against Children identified legal prohibition of all violence against children including HTP.[36]

Transsocietal (Global) Violence

Emerging transsocietal changes present new existential threats to children. These evolving realities require new conceptual frameworks, approaches, and a willingness of professionals to confront the accelerating challenges the world's children are facing.

War and armed conflict

Millions of children live with armed conflict, and nearly 33% of them live outside their country of birth as refugees.[37] Children are caught in the crossfire or are directly targeted by combatants, resulting in injury, illness, disability, psychological trauma, and death.[38] Forced displacement, separation from family, and the destruction of health, education, and economic infrastructure leads to a broad range of adverse effects.[39] Children are recruited and forced into armed groups, with devastating consequences for their health and long-term functioning.[40]

Child rights
- CRC Article 38 requests all governments to respect international humanitarian law to protect children. This includes refraining from recruiting children younger than 15 years.
- The Optional Protocol to the CRC on the Involvement of Children in Armed Conflict was adopted in 2000 to strengthen the protection of children.[41]
- The Geneva Conventions also speak to the special need to protect children during conflict and war.[42]

Children on the move

The magnitude of international migration has grown at an unprecedented rate reaching a level of 258 million persons in 2017.[43] Since the turn of the twenty-first century, 50 million children worldwide have crossed international borders with another 17 million internally displaced.[44] In 2018 children younger than 18 years constitute more than half of the 26 million refugees worldwide.[45] Migration is associated with trauma and violence including physical and sexual abuse, abduction, trafficking, and other travails throughout their journeys.[46]

Child rights
- CRC, Article 22 requires governments to ensure that refugee children or those seeking asylum are protected and receive humanitarian assistance.

Globalization

The world's children are at great risk from the impact of globalization. Globalization is defined as, "the interconnection and interdependence among countries manifested through international economic, political, and social networks."[47] It can negatively affect child health through increased influence of high-income countries, privatization, and international trade agreements.[48]

Child rights

- The United Nations is considering the establishment of a commission of CRC signatories, World Bank, UNICEF, and the High Commissioner for Human Rights to formulate a plan addressing globalization's impact on children.[49]

Climate change

Children are disproportionately affected by climate change, particularly indigenous children, children living in poverty, those with developmental disabilities, and children displaced by conflict.[50] The impact is magnified because countries most susceptible to climate change have a higher proportion of children.[51] Climate change has increased the frequency and intensity of extreme weather events. This negatively affects access to food, water, and health services. It is estimated that currently 160 million children live in areas at risk of drought and 500 million live in flood zones—both of which decrease accessibility to safe water and adequate food—these are also populations most likely to be displaced with attendant risks and consequences.

Child rights

- CRC, Article 6 recognizes that every child has the inherent right to life and optimal survival and development, which is now under threat due to climate change.
- CRC, Article 24 articulates the child's right to health care, water, nutritious food, and a safe and clean environment.

RESPONSES NEEDED TO END VIOLENCE AGAINST CHILDREN

Violence affects more than 1 billion children annually.[52] In 2017, the report on *Ending Violence in Childhood* detailed the causes and consequences of childhood violence and identified evidence-based strategies to prevent it.[53]

Clinical Response

Responses at the clinical level will require training and resource development, such that all agencies interacting with children are well poised to respond to all forms of VAC.

Attention should be focused on enhancing capacity in the following areas:

- All child and youth providers should be trained in a trauma-informed approach to care that recognizes and responds to trauma in a manner that is open, collaborative, and nonjudgmental.
- All professional and community health workers must be trained to recognize, report, and respond to VAC in accordance with their local jurisdictions and legislative frameworks.
- Mental and behavioral health services must be available.
- Rights respecting "safe zones" supported by trained caring adults should be established in conflict zones to mitigate the impact of VAC.
- Children and youth must be educated about their rights with activities developed to promote respect, self-confidence, and empowerment.

Systems-Based Response

A systems-based response is critical to ensure resources are available to mitigate the impact of VAC. Community engagement to identify, report, and respond to VAC involves collaboration among stakeholders.

- Agencies must educate themselves and promote awareness of the many forms of VAC and monitor their own systems for violations.

- Juvenile justice systems require oversight to ensure that youth are afforded adequate living conditions and are free of torture and deprivation. In addition, while being held in detention, rights must always be respected and all measures taken to optimize the growth and development of youth in custody.
- Individuals with disabilities require special protections to ensure their safety and well-being. Communities must implement programming to ensure this need is met.
- Resources should be allocated to social programming to prevent VAC and mitigate the harms of VAC through evidence-based practices.

Policy Response

From a policy perspective there is much work to be done in ensuring global implementation of international humanitarian laws, as well as ongoing collaboration across countries to ensure the protection of the world's most valuable asset—our children and youth.

- The Sustainable Development Goals provide a framework to end global poverty and optimize health and well-being across the globe. Implementing these goals will address many of the root causes for VAC.
- Promote the Global Initiative to End All Corporal Punishment of Children.
- Eliminate traditional practices that harm girls and women, including forced child marriage and female genital mutilation.
- Advocate to end child labor practices and promote of educational opportunity.
- Abolish all forms of child trafficking through national, bilateral, and multinational collaboratives.
- International awareness to address the causes of displaced children is growing. In 2018, the International Conference to Adopt the Global Compact for Safe, Orderly, and Regular Migration and the Compact on Refugees were finalized.[54,55] The Compacts provide a global human rights framework to support global efforts to address this crisis.

It is critically important that the impact of globalization and climate change be acknowledged with new policies to mitigate their ongoing impact on children.

SUMMARY

We must reconceptualize the concept of CAN as VAC, acknowledge the global scope of violence against children, and frame it in terms of child rights. The principle of interdependence demands all protection, promotion, and participation rights must be fulfilled for all children to prevent and mitigate the effects of VAC. The principle of accountability requires all pediatric health professionals be duty-bearers for fulfilling the rights of all children. To ensure optimal survival and development without discrimination, VAC in all its manifestations must be addressed using the parlance, principles, standards, and norms of child rights.

DISCLOSURE

The authors have nothing to disclose.

REFERENCES

1. Reading R, Bissell S, Goldhagen J, et al. Promotion of children's rights and prevention of child maltreatment. Lancet 2009;373(9660):332–43.

2. WHO. (2002). World report on violence and health. Geneva. WHO Global Consultation on Violence and Health. Violence: a public health priority. Geneva (Switzerland): World Health Organization; 1996.

3. Article 19: protection from abuse and neglect. child rights international network. Available at: https://archive.crin.org/en/home/rights/convention/articles/article-19-protection-abuse-and-neglect.html. Accessed July 26, 2020.

4. Report of the independent expert for the United Nations study on violence against children. August 29, 2006. Available at: https://documents-dds-ny.un.org/doc/UNDOC/GEN/N06/491/05/PDF/N0649105.pdf?OpenElement. Accessed July 26, 2020.

5. UN sustainable development goals knowledge platform violence against children. Available at: https://sustainabledevelopment.un.org/topics/violenceagainstchildren. Accessed July 26, 2020.

6. Svevo-Cianci KA, Herzog M, Krappman L, et al. The new UN CRC general comment 13-The rights of "The child to freedom from all forms of violence"—changing how the world conceptualizes child protection. Child Abuse Negl 2011;3:979–89.

7. Goldhagen J, Shenoda S, Oberg C, et al. Justice and equity: a global agenda for child health and well-being. Lancet 2010. https://doi.org/10.1016/S2352-4642(19)30346-3.

8. Bronfenbrenner U. Developmental research, public policy and the ecology of childhood. Child Dev 1974;45:1–5.

9. Raman S, Kadir A, Seth R, et al. Violence against children of the world-burden, consequences and recommendations for action. 2017. Available at: https://www.issop.org/category/contents/issop-position-statements/page/3/. Accessed July 26, 2020.

10. Kempe CH, Silverman FN, Steele BF, et al. The battered-child syndrome. JAMA 1962;181(1):17–24.

11. Butchart A, Harvey AP, Mian M, et al. Preventing child maltreatment: a guide to taking action and generating evidence. 2006. Available at: https://www.who.int/violence_injury_prevention/publications/violence/child_maltreatment/en/. Accessed January 19, 2021.

12. Finkelhor D, Ormrod RK, Turner HA. Re-victimization patterns in a national longitudinal sample of children and youth. Child Abuse Negl 2007;31:479–502.

13. Jones L, Bellis MA, Wood S, et al. (2012). Prevalence and risk of violence against children with disabilities: a systematic review and meta-analysis of observational studies. Lancet 2012;380:899–907.

14. MacMillan HL, Wathen CN, Varcoe CM. (2013). Intimate partner violence in the family: Considerations for children's safety. Child Abuse Negl 2013;37:1186–91.

15. Thackeray JD, Randell KA. Epidemiology of intimate partner violence. child abuse and neglect: diagnosis, treatment and evidence. 2011. p. 23-27. Available at https://corescholar.libraries.wright.edu/pediatrics/470/. Accessed January 19, 2021.

16. Knox M. On hitting children: a review of corporal punishment in the United States. J Pediatr Health Care 2010;24:103–7.

17. Initiative to End All Corporal Punishment of Children. (2017). Available at: http://www.endcorporalpunishment.org/. Accessed July 27, 2020.

18. Portela MJO, Pells K. Corporal punishment in schools longitudinal evidence from Ethiopia, India, Peru and Viet Nam. Florence (Italy): UNICEF Office of Research – Innocenti; 2015.

19. Committee on the rights of the child (2011) General Comments No. 13 'Article 19; The right of the children to freedom from all forms of violence". Available at: www.crin.org/docs/CRC.C.GC.13_en_AUV-1.pdf. Accessed July 26, 2020.

20. Olweus D. Bullying at school: basic facts and effects of a school based intervention program. J Child Psychol Psychiatry 1994;35:1171–90.

21. Pinheiro PS. World report on violence against children. 2006. Available at https://digitallibrary.un.org/record/587334?ln=en. Accessed January 19, 2021.

22. Bullying and Human Rights, Rights Sites News, Promoting Hum Rights Education Classroom, 2010;6:1–10. Available at: https://www.theadvocatesforhumanrights.org/uploads/rights_sites_bullying.pdf. Accessed January 19, 2021.

23. Kurek N, Darzi LA, Maa J. A worldwide perspective provides insights into why a US Surgeon General Annual Report on firearm injuries is needed in America. Curr Trauma Rep 2020;6:36–43.

24. Cunningham RM, Carter PM, Zimmerman M. The firearm safety among children and teens (FACTS) Consortium: defining the current state of the science on pediatric firearm injury prevention. J Behav Med 2019;42:702–5.

25. The impact of gun violence on children and teens. Everytown Research & Policy Fact Sheet, May 29, 2019. Available at: https://everytownresearch.org/report/the-impact-of-gun-violence-on-children-and-teens/.

26. ILO. (2017). Child labour. Available at: http://www.ilo.org/global/topics/child-labour/lang–en/index.htm. Accessed July 26, 2020.

27. UNICEF. (2005). Combatting child trafficking. Available at: https://www.unicef.org/publications/files/IPU_combattingchildtrafficking_GB(1).pdf. Accessed July 26, 2020.

28. Pais MS. The protection of children from sexual exploitation optional protocol to the convention on the rights of the child on the sale of children, child prostitution and child pornography. The International Journal or Children's Rights 2010;18:551–66. Available at: https://brill.com/view/journals/chil/18/4/article-p551_6.xml.

29. Pinheiro PS. World report on violence against children. Geneva (Switzerland): Office of the High Commissioner for Human Rights (OHCHR), the United Nations Children's Fund (UNICEF) and the World Health Organization (WHO); 2006.

30. Jenney A. Keeping children safe from violence: strengthening child protection systems in their accountability to identify, refer and respond to cases of violence against children. Geneva(Switzerland): UNICEF; 2013.

31. Owen M, Goldhagen J. Children and solitary confinement: a call to action. Pediatrics 2016;137(5):e20154180.

32. Stalker K, McArthur K. Child abuse, child protection and disabled children: a review of recent research. Child Abuse Review 2012;21(1):24–40. Available at: https://onlinelibrary.wiley.com/doi/abs/10.1002/car.1154.

33. International NGO council on violence against children. Violating children's rights: harmful practices based on tradition, culture, religion or superstition. New York (NY): 2012. Available at: https://resourcecentre.savethechildren.net/node/7212/pdf/7212.pdf. Accessed January 19, 2021.

34. Boyden J, Pankhurst A, Tafere Y. Child protection and harmful traditional practices: female early marriage and genital modification in Ethiopia. Dev Pract 2012;22(4):510–22.

35. Winter B, Thompson D, Jeffreys S. The UN approach to harmful traditional practices. Int Fem J Polit 2002;4:72–94.

36. UN Special Representative of the Secretary-General on Violence Against Children. Protecting children from harmful practices in plural legal systems-with

special emphasis on Africa. 2012. Available at: https://violenceagainstchildren. un.org/news/protecting-children-harmful-practices-plural-legal-systems-special-emphasis-africa-0.

37. UNICEF. More than 1 in 10 children living in countries and areas affected by armed conflict. New York (NY): United States Fund for UNICEF; 2015.

38. Shenoda S, Kadir A, Pitterman S, et al. The effects of armed conflict on children. Pediatrics 2018;142(6):e20182585.

39. Feder M, Choonara I. (2012). Armed conflict and child health. Arch Dis Child 2012;97:59–62.

40. Betancourt TS, Borisova I, Williams TP, et al. Research review: psychosocial adjustment and mental health in former child soldiers. J Child Psychol Psychiatry 2013;54:17–36.

41. Helle D. Optional protocol on the involvement of children in armed conflict to the convention on the rights of the child. International Review of the Red Cross 82:797–823. Available at: https://www.cambridge.org/core/journals/international-review-of-the-red-cross/article/abs/optional-protocol-on-the-involvement-of-child ren-in-armed-conflict-to-the-convention-on-the-rights-of-the-child/6FC9B7FA36C 67903EC7BA65DCD4D2BE9.

42. Fonseka B. The protection of child soldiers in International Law. Asia Pac J Hum Right Law 2001;2:69–89.

43. United Nations, Department of Economic and Social Affairs, Population Division. Trends in international migrant stock: the 2017 revision migrants by age and sex. New York (NY): United Nations; 2017.

44. Uprooted-The Growing Crisis for Refugee & Migrant Children. UNICEF, September 2016. Available at: http://www.unicef.org/publications/index_92710. html. Accessed July 26, 2020.

45. UNHCR. Global trends: forced displacement in 2018. Geneva (Switzerland): 2019. Available at: https://www.unhcr.org/5ee200e37.pdf. Accessed January 19, 2021.

46. Oberg CN. The arc of migration and the impact on children's health and well-being. Children 2019;6:100.

47. Lee K. Globalization: what is it and how does it affect health? Med J Aust 2004; 180:156–8.

48. Wamala S. The impact of globalization on maternal and child health. In: Ehiri J, editor. Maternal and child health: global challenges, programs, and policies. Springer; 2009. p. 135-49. Available at: https://link.springer.com/chapter/10. 1007%2Fb106524_8. Accessed January 19, 2021.

49. Harnessing globalization for children: a report to UNICEF. Available at: https:// www.unicef-irc.org/research/ESP/globalization/. Accessed July 26, 2020.

50. Ebi K, Paulson JA. Climate change and children. Pediatr Clin North Am 2007;54: 213–26.

51. Analytical study on the relationship between climate change and the full and effective enjoyment of the rights of the child, (A/HRC/35/13). United Nations Human Rights-Office of the High Commissioner.

52. Hillis S, Mercy J, Amobi A, et al. Global prevalence of past-year violence against children: a systematic review and minimum estimates. Pediatrics 2016; 137(3):1–22.

53. Know violence in childhood. Ending violence in childhood. global report 2017 New Delhi, India: know violence in childhood, 2017. 2017. Available at: http:// globalreport.knowviolenceinchildhood.org/. Accessed January 19, 2021.

54. UN Refugees and Migrants. Global compact for safe, orderly and regular migration. 2018. Available at: https://www.un.org/pga/72/wp-content/uploads/sites/51/2018/07/180713_Agreed-Outcome_Global-Compact-for-Migration.pdf. Accessed July 26, 2020.
55. Refugees UN, Migrants. Global compact on refugees. 2019. Available at: https://www.unhcr.org/ph/the-global-compact-on-refugees. Accessed July 26, 2020.

Case Studies and Discussions

Forcible Displacement, Migration, and Violence Against Children and Families in Latin America

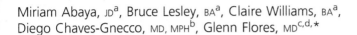

Miriam Abaya, JD[a], Bruce Lesley, BA[a], Claire Williams, BA[a],
Diego Chaves-Gnecco, MD, MPH[b], Glenn Flores, MD[c,d,*]

KEYWORDS

- Forced displacement • Immigration • Children • Families • Best interests • Policy
- Latinos

KEY POINTS

- Latin American families face high levels of violence, gender violence, poverty, extortion, corruption, and climate change in their home countries, forcing them to flee to the United States.
- The US immigration system has not shifted from a deterrence model, despite the increase in immigrant families arriving at the southern border and living in the United States.
- US government policies enacted between 2016 and 2020 have harmed children by returning them and their families to violence; traumatizing them through detention and family separation; denying them access to benefits that would support their health, emotional well-being, and financial stability; and leaving them with lifelong consequences due to toxic stress.
- US immigration policies must be governed by the best-interests-of-the-child standard to be child-centered and protective of children and families.

[a] First Focus on Children, 1400 "Eye" Street Northwest, Suite 650, Washington, DC 20005, USA; [b] Salud Para Niños Program, Department of Pediatrics, UPMC Children's Hospital of Pittsburgh, University of Pittsburgh School of Medicine, 3420 Fifth Avenue/Euler Way, Pittsburgh, PA 15213, USA; [c] Health Services Research Institute, Connecticut Children's Medical Center, Department of Pediatrics, University of Connecticut School of Medicine, 282 Washington Street, Hartford, CT 06106, USA; [d] Department of Pediatrics, University of Miami Miller School of Medicine, Holtz Children's Hospital, 1601 Northwest 12th Avenue, Miami, FL 33137, USA
* Corresponding author. Department of Pediatrics, University of Miami Miller School of Medicine, 1601 NW 12th Avenue, 9th Floor, Miami, FL 33136.
E-mail address: gl9flores@gmail.com

Pediatr Clin N Am 68 (2021) 371–387
https://doi.org/10.1016/j.pcl.2020.12.003
0031-3955/21/© 2020 Elsevier Inc. All rights reserved.
pediatric.theclinics.com

INTRODUCTION

Forcible Displacement of Latin American Children and Their Families Owing to Violence

At the end of 2019, the number of forcibly displaced people reached almost 80 million people—a record high. Of this number, almost 29 million were refugees or asylum seekers, one-half of them children fleeing persecution and violence.[1,2] Latin America is no different; growing numbers of children and families have fled the Northern Triangle and Venezuela in the past few years.

The following real-life case and those recounted elsewhere in this article illustrate the challenges faced by children and families who have fled violence in their countries of origin (initials are used to maintain anonymity):

> M.M., a single mother of 3 children from rural El Salvador, was forced to escape to the United States after gangs started threatening J.M., her teenage son. In Central America, and in particular in El Salvador, gangs act as criminal organizations. One of these gangs demanded money from J.M. If he refused to comply, they vowed to kidnap him or kill his mother. Realizing it was no longer safe for the family to live in El Salvador, M.M. made the difficult decision to immigrate to the United States. After M.M. and her children departed, the gang began harassing M.M.'s remaining family members, extorting them for money in return for "protection." M.M.'s brother, C.M., became the gang's new target, and they demanded payment from him, as they had with J.M. C.M. refused to contribute to an organization that instills fear and intimidates the Salvadoran people. For that, he paid with his life.

The United Nations High Commissioner for Refugees has documented a notable increase in asylum seekers from Mexico and Central America in recent years. These are people who are seeking refugee status—protection from persecution based on a protected ground—but whose claims have not yet been determined.[3] From 2012 to mid-

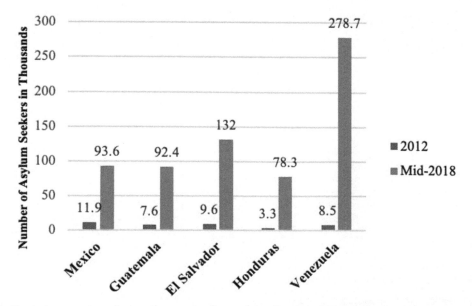

Fig. 1. Increase in asylum seekers and refugees from 2012 to mid-2018. (Data source: Center for American Progress.[4])

2018, asylum-seeker populations increased by 686% in Mexico, 2272% in Honduras, 1275% in El Salvador, 1115% in Guatemala, and 3179% in Venezuela (**Fig. 1**).[4] Widespread instability in Mexico and Central and South America has increased the number of children and their families seeking asylum in the United States in recent years. During the 2019 fiscal year, more than 6000 individuals from Mexico, 185,000 from Guatemala, 56,000 from El Salvador, and 188,000 from Honduras were apprehended with a family member by the US Customs and Border Protection (CBP) at the southern border.[5] Unlike active war zones, there is no single, overarching reason for mass family migration from Mexico, Central America, and South America. The exodus of children and families, instead, derives from an agglomeration of social, political, and economic factors, including violence, organized crime, poverty, corruption, and climate change.

Violence

Certain Central American countries are plagued by widespread violence and are widely considered to be some of the most dangerous regions in the world. In 2018, homicide rates were 26 per 100,000 people in Mexico, 22 per 100,000 in Guatemala, 40 per 100,000 in Honduras, and 51 per 100,00 in El Salvador.[6] Although Venezuela does not release official crime statistics, it is estimated that the rate of violent deaths was 81 per 100,000 inhabitants in 2018.[7] For contrast, one of the safest countries within the region, Costa Rica, had a homicide rate of 12 per 100,000.[6] Additionally, comparison with homicide rates in the United States reveals why these families flee to our southern border. The highest US homicide rates are in Mississippi, Louisiana, and the District of Columbia, with rates of 13.4 per 100,000, 13.3 per 100,000, and 19.01 per 100,000, respectively. Rates are even lower in California (4.8/100,000), Florida (6.6/100,000), New York (3.2/100,000), and Texas (5.4/100,000), the states where most immigrants resettle in the United States.[7] Everything considered, the dangers that families with children face in their home countries prove too great for them, forcing them to journey north in search of a safe place to raise a family.

Violence owing to narcotics dealing and trafficking is quite prevalent in Mexico and certain Central American countries. The Northern Triangle, composed of Guatemala, El Salvador, and Honduras, is situated in the middle of the main drug shipment route from South America to the United States, and is where cartel-affiliated groups act as *transportistas*, who oversee the movement of narcotics across the region. Many families find themselves in the cross-fire of drug deals and/or gang turf wars in both Mexico and the Northern Triangle, which has grave consequences, even for innocent bystanders. For example, a relative of M.M., the woman described in the case presented elsewhere in this article, was brutally murdered after he witnessed the local gang kill a police officer in the streets. In Mexico, a country dominated by transnational criminal organizations, roughly 150,000 murders can be attributed to organized crime, out of 288,000 intentional homicides reported since 2006.[8] Murder is the most extreme version of violence against individuals in Mexico and Central and South America, but other crimes, such as assault, robberies, and domestic violence, are rampant. Because criminal groups control many areas in the region, innocent children and families often get caught in the cross-fire.

Gender violence

These regions also are considered some of the most dangerous in the world for girls and women. Even as homicide rates decrease, femicide—the killing of girls and women for gender-related reasons—is increasing. El Salvador's 2016 murder rate per 100,000 women was 10.2, the worst worldwide.[6] Honduras recorded 5.8 murders per 100,000 women in 2016, and Guatemala had more than 2 murders per 100,000 women in 2017.[9] In Mexico, femicides have increased by 145% in the past 15 years.[10] These killings tend to result from domestic violence, divorce, and verbal altercations. Girls and women of all ages in both Mexico and Central and South America are frequent targets of gender-based violence and sexual violence. Girls and women in these regions are often powerless against their aggressors, and the legal systems rarely support their pleas for fairness under the law. In a place where women can be killed for simply being a woman, many girls and women flee out of fear for their safety.

Other challenges: poverty, extortion, corruption, and climate change
In addition to violence, other factors threaten the daily safety and well-being of families in these regions, such as cyclical poverty, extortion, corruption, and climate change. In 2018, more than one-half of Mexico's and Central America's populations lived in poverty.[11] Members of gangs and cartel groups enter the criminal market out of desperation for higher wages, but their illicit activity actually furthers the cycle of economic depravity in the region. Extortion, the process of obtaining money through force or threats, as seen in J.M.'s case, is intimately linked to poverty and insecurity, which encourages families to migrate. Sums expected by criminal groups often exceed individuals' ability to pay, so many families like M.M.'s are forced to escape to countries where funding criminal groups is not required to conduct business or live peacefully.

Criminal groups also may buy the goodwill of political and law enforcement authorities in Mexico and certain Central and South American countries. When people entrusted with protecting everyday citizens are on criminals' payrolls, high levels of corruption and impunity reign. Transparency International's Corruption Perceptions Index, the world's most used indicator of corruption, ranks countries on a scale of 0 (very corrupt) to 100 (very clean). Mexico, Guatemala, El Salvador, Honduras, and Venezuela's Corruption Perceptions Index scores are 29, 26, 34, 26, and 16, respectively.[12]

Climate change has emerged as an increasingly important driver of migration in recent years. Prolonged droughts limit crop harvests and result in decreased wages and unemployment for families who depend on agriculture to survive. The Northern Triangle falls within the Central American Dry Corridor, a tropical dry forest in western Central America that is one of the world's most vulnerable regions to climate change. By 2030, Mexico's cropland suitability will likely decrease by 40% to 70%, which will mean more forced displacements of families as their livelihoods become unsustainable.[13] Heightened competition for limited resources may increase violence in a region already plagued by organized crime and economic deprivation.

Conclusions
The mountain of obstacles facing Mexican and Central and South American families in the region often proves too difficult to overcome. Analyzing the situation on the ground in Mexico and Central and South America makes it clear why children and families emigrate. They worry for their health and safety, they are overwhelmed by senseless violence, they yearn for economic freedom, and they hope to live without fear. Understanding why thousands upon thousands of families are fleeing from these regions is a key first step to creating policy that addresses the needs of these children in families when they arrive in the United States.

THE ASYLUM PROCESS FOR FAMILIES

In 2014, the demographics of migrants arriving at the southern US border started to shift from Mexican single adults to children and families from El Salvador, Guatemala, and Honduras.[14] In 2018, the number of children and families arriving annually had increased 4-fold, compared with 2013.[14] Nevertheless, US immigration law and policy have maintained "prevention through deterrence" policies, rather than transitioning to policies that would protect and support children and families.

At the Border

Under US and international law, the United States is prohibited from turning away anyone seeking protection from persecution or torture at its southern border, whether protection is sought at a port of entry or after crossing without authorization.[15] When families request asylum from CBP at the border, they are taken to border facilities to be processed and interviewed by an asylum officer to prove that they are likely to face persecution if returned to their country.[16] If an asylum officer finds that an asylum seeker has a significant possibility of being granted asylum or another form of protection, the seeker and their family are then referred to immigration court to go through regular immigration proceedings before an immigration judge. If they do not, they can be removed from the border.[16]

Under CBP's own policies, immigrant families should spend no longer than 72 hours in CBP custody[17] because border facilities are built for short-term processing. Border holding cells are often referred to as *hieleras* (Spanish for freezers or ice boxes) by those who spend time there: they are cold rooms with concrete benches and no beds.[18] Although children and families now account for most of those arriving at the border, these facilities have not been renovated to be more humane or welcoming.

Applying for Asylum

Families passing their credible-fear interview are either released or transferred to detention. When the government decides to detain families, they are transferred to 1 of 3 family detention facilities run by Immigration and Customs Enforcement (ICE).[19] Families may also be released directly from CBP custody on parole to live with a sponsor in the community.[14]

At their final destination, families continue their asylum claims before an immigration judge. Under international and US law, individuals establish asylum if they show that they suffered persecution or have a well-founded fear of future persecution based on their race, religion, nationality, political opinion, or membership in a particular social group.[20] Children in families can be a derivative beneficiary of their parent's asylum application, meaning that they will get asylum if their parent's claim is granted.[21]

The asylum process can take years to conclude. If families do not receive a grant of asylum after years of waiting, ICE might come into their home or community to arrest the family and deport them. If, however, the primary applicant—usually the parent— convinces an immigration judge that they have suffered or have a well-founded fear of persecution based on protected grounds, they and their derivative beneficiaries will receive asylum.

Families' Access to Benefits

While asylum seekers await a final decision on their asylum claim, they can apply for work authorization.[16] The lengthy time period between the application for asylum and the final decision, however, can leave families in uncertainty over their health, emotional well-being, and economic support.

Once individuals are granted asylum, they and their family are eligible to apply for a Green Card 1 year after the asylum decision.[22] Immigrants receiving Green Cards, however, must wait 5 years before being eligible for federal benefits, such as Medicaid, the Children's Health Insurance Program, and Temporary Assistance for

Needy Families.[23] Additionally, undocumented immigrants are excluded from the narrow category of immigrants who qualify for federal assistance.[23]

DISCUSSION

Children and families who are forcibly displaced owing to violence face many threats to their safety in their home countries. US policy vis-à-vis the treatment of such displaced families and children has garnered a great deal of criticism nationally and globally owing to the inhuman conditions and overall lack of due process in the consideration of current requests for asylum. Moreover, the government has not had a legal mandate to consider the best interests—the safety and well-being—of immigrant children, including children in families (ie, with parents or legal guardians). Between 2016 and 2020, the US government has put in place policies that harm children and families seeking protection, making it more difficult for them to receive protection in the United States and support once they are able to remain in the United States.

Unaccompanied children (children <18 years old, without legal status, and with no parent or legal guardian to care for them)[24] coming to the United States have few of the vital protections they need regarding their care, custody, and due process.[25,26] The protections they do have do not address all the needs of unaccompanied children, and not all protections extend to children with a parent or legal guardian. As a result of such gaps in protections and government policies enacted between 2016 and 2020, children in immigrant families do not have the protection and support they need to ensure their health and well-being as they seek safety in the United States and attempt to grow and thrive in their communities. Without protective and child-centered policies, immigrant children and families face harm and detrimental effects at every stage of seeking protection in the United States—from the border to their life in their new communities.

Border and Asylum Policies Harm Children and Return Families to Violence

US border policies, including many of those enacted between 2016 and 2020, have put children directly in harm's way. In 2018, the US government implemented the practice of "metering"—limiting the number of people who could approach the border to seek asylum per day, forcing children and families to wait in Mexico without basic amenities and as targets of violence.[27] In January 2019, the US government implemented the so-called Migrant Protection Protocols, otherwise known as the Remain in Mexico Program.[28] Similar to the 1990s US government program that removed Haitian asylum seekers to Guantanamo Bay to determine their asylum status,[29] asylum seekers arriving at the border are forced to return to Mexico to await immigration proceedings, rather than waiting in the United States. As of May 2020, more than 65,000 people were forced to return to Mexico, including 16,000 children and nearly 500 infants.[28] These families live in makeshift camps on the border and have hearings in tent courts with immigration judges who hear their stories of persecution by video.[30] Because of the dangerous conditions in Mexico, many families make the impossible choice to send their children to the border alone to receive protection as unaccompanied children.[28,31]

Metering and Remain in Mexico force families back to dangerous Mexican border communities where cartels target migrants. Human Rights First has compiled at least 1114 publicly reported cases of murder, rape, torture, kidnapping, and other acts of violence against asylum seekers in the Remain in Mexico Program, including 265 children who were kidnapped or nearly kidnapped.[28]

Reports indicate that the US government approaches propagated inadequate conditions in CBP facilities to deter families from seeking protection in the United States. The inappropriate nature of CBP facilities came to the forefront of national news in the summer of 2019, when increasing numbers of children and families arrived at the border. CBP held children and families in metal cages and cold cells for prolonged periods—with some children held in such conditions for up to 1 month.[32] CBP failed to provide basic hygiene products, such as soap, toothbrushes, and toothpaste, to those in their custody.[32] Migrants who arrived with health conditions were unable to access medical care.[33] Six children died in 8 months in CBP custody, 3 of whom were children with their families.[34]

The RZ family are young parents from Mexico who fled gang extortion. Fearing for their safety, the family decided to leave for the United States. Mrs. RZ's mother had been living in the United States for the last 20 years, and the RZ family planned to live with her. While crossing the border, Mr. and Mrs. RZ were separated. Mrs. RZ was held at the border for 2 months while she was pregnant, before she was released and able to reunite with her mother.

The United States has also targeted access to asylum. In 2019, the United States implemented an asylum transit ban, which barred people from receiving asylum if they passed through another country on their journey to the United States.[35] In June 2020, the Administration published a proposed rule that would make it almost impossible for families from Central America to receive asylum by denying asylum based on the exact types of violence that many Central American families are fleeing, such as gang violence or domestic violence.[36]

The United States' current (2020) regressive asylum policies have 1 extremely likely result—returning children and families to the danger they fled.[35] Because many families must pass through other countries to arrive at the US border, they are barred from seeking asylum under the transit ban, regardless of whether they would meet the standards to prove they fear persecution in their country of origin. The asylum rule published in June 2020[36] could change the US asylum system forever, bringing the United States out of line with global asylum standards and denying asylum to many people from Central America. These changes mean that families will go through the lengthy and complex immigration process only to be denied asylum and returned to the same communities where they faced violence before their journey.

The US government has used the novel coronavirus disease-2019 (COVID-19) pandemic as a cover for even more harmful border policies. On March 20, 2020, the Centers for Disease Control and Prevention published an order that shut down the border between Mexico and the United States for any "nonessential" travel, with no exception for asylum seekers, including families and children.[37] As a result, almost 200,000 people have been expelled at the border—either returned to Mexico or put on flights back to their home country—without any consideration of their safety or fear of persecution.[37,38] Some children and families were held in hotels with an ICE contractor for long periods before being forcibly returned to their home country.[39] Dozens of public health officials have called the public health rationale for the order "specious," and have provided measures to process asylum seekers at the border safely.[40,41] Nevertheless, these expulsions continue.

Detention Is Never in the Best Interests of Children

The federal government argues that they have the right to detain asylum seekers, including families, while their asylum claim is pending, and has expanded family detention as the number of families arriving at the border increases.[16] In response to criticism from advocates and public health experts, the Obama Administration implemented the Family Case Management Program, in which families resided in the community, met with case managers, had a mandatory orientation program about the immigration process, and were referred to legal, social, and educational services in their community.[42] Based on an evaluation by the Women's Refugee Commission, the Family Case Management Program, although not perfect, had good outcomes—99% of families complied with their court hearings and ICE check-ins, and more than one-half of families had legal representation.[42] Additionally, ICE historically had a policy of "safe release" from the border, where they coordinated the necessary plans for asylum-seeking families to travel to their sponsor's residence.[14]

The current (2020) administration's policies, however, have favored the detention of children and families, rather than their release. By 2018, the Family Case Management Program had been terminated, thereby ending safe release at the border and continuing the detention of families.[14,42] During the COVID-19 pandemic, the administration has refused to release the remaining families, including 120 children in detention, despite a federal judge characterizing these facilities as being "on fire" with the virus.[43] As of August 2020, close to 100 people in these facilities have tested positive for COVID-19.[43]

Studies and reports have documented that detention substantially harms children. Parents report that, while in detention, their children developmentally regress and suffer from loss of appetite, sleep disturbances, clinginess, withdrawal, and aggression.[44] Parents also exhibit depression, anxiety, and hopelessness.[45] This toxic stress for both parents and children results in strained parent–child relationships.[41] In evaluating the impact of detention for children, the American Academy of Pediatrics stated that "there is no evidence indicating that any time in detention is safe for children."[46]

Family detention also impacts family access to protection in the United States because detention facilities are mostly located in small or rural cities, far from immigration courts and organizations that can provide legal representation.[47] Additionally, families in detention appear at their immigration hearings by video.[47] Compounding the complicated nature of immigration law with a lack of representation, video hearings, and the adverse effects of detention, it is not surprising that detained families are more likely to lose their asylum cases and return to face the dangers they are fleeing.[47]

Family Separation Inflicts Lifelong Trauma

In the summer of 2017, the US government began its policy of family separation to discourage families from coming to the United States, formalizing the practice in its "zero-tolerance policy" in the summer of 2018.[48] As a result of that program, more than 5400 children were separated from their parents.[49] Although the administration ended the zero-tolerance policy as mandated by a court order, separations still continue based on parents' alleged criminal history or unfitness, without any safeguards or processes for reunification.[50] To this day, 545 children remain separated from parents who cannot be located.[51]

The family separation policy intentionally imposed harm and trauma on children. During Zero Tolerance, government officials lied to families and children, failed to document and keep track of children and their caregivers within and between agencies that are entrusted with their protection, and refused to comply with court orders to end family separations and improve the protections of children. The results were, and are, significant trauma, toxic stress, and life-long harm to thousands of innocent children, 40% of whom were less than 10 years old.[52]

Physicians for Human Rights surveyed 17 adults and 9 children who were separated during Zero Tolerance.[52] They found that the policy met the criteria for torture, given the traumatic responses exhibited by the children and their caregivers. Clinicians who interviewed families noted that children who suffered separation exhibited signs of regression, nightmares, and other sleeping difficulties; frequent crying; and aggression. Several clinicians pointed out that many children and their caregivers met the diagnostic criteria for post-traumatic stress disorder, major depressive disorder, or generalized anxiety disorder. These trauma responses, and additional deleterious consequences for financial stability, occur for families separated by ICE during enforcement actions in communities.[53] Physicians for Human Rights noted that, for recovery from trauma, families required "psychiatric and behavioral health interventions in the context of strong social and family-mediated support."[52]

Exclusion from Benefits Results in Negative Impacts on Health, Emotional Well-Being, and Economic Stability

Even for families who gain some form of permanency in the United States, there remain barriers to services that would improve their health, well-being, and stability. The US government has lengthened the time that asylum seekers must wait for work authorization, which undermines the ability of families to care for themselves and their children.[54]

The US government has enacted policy changes that deter immigrants from accessing public benefits for which they may be eligible. In February 2020, the US government finalized changes to the public-charge admissibility test, which is a policy that would deny someone a green card if the government determines that they may depend on government benefits as their main source of support in the future.[55] Changes to the policy expand the benefits that might count against immigrants in their application for a Green Card to include supports like Medicaid (excluding children <21 years old), Temporary Assistance for Needy Families, Supplemental Nutrition Assistance Program, and federal housing assistance.[56] Although the rule only applies to a narrow group of immigrants, it has had a chilling effect: many immigrant families have opted out of accessing benefits for which they are eligible for fear of negative consequences to their immigration status.[56]

Evidence shows that because of these US laws delaying or excluding immigrants from access to benefits, immigrants tend to support their families with low-paying jobs that do not provide health insurance.[57] Children in immigrant families suffer from higher rates of child poverty and food insecurity.[57] Immigrant women and children are less likely to use health services, resulting in poorer health and health care outcomes.[57]

The RD family fled threats from paramilitary groups in Venezuela and are seeking asylum in the United States. During an evaluation from a local free pediatric clinic before starting school, the youngest child was found to have a congenital cataract, which had caused him to live with a visual deficit for his whole life. Owing to the lack of health insurance, the necessary treatment had to wait. Fortunately, Mr. RD found a job with health insurance for the entire family, and the young child was able to get treatment at the local children's hospital. Without the free clinic to diagnose the child's condition and without a job providing health insurance, the young child might have continued to wait years for treatment, with the potential for a worsening of the visual deficits.

During the COVID-19 pandemic, families still face barriers to accessing public benefits. Mixed-status families have been excluded from legislative COVID-19 relief packages and cannot receive Medicaid for COVID-19 treatment or the cash payments distributed to other families. These families' exclusion affects 15.4 million people, including 3.7 million US citizen and green card-holding children.[58]

Recommendations

When it comes to immigration policies impacting the lives of children, policy solutions should be governed by a best-interest-of-the-child standards. The best interests of the child is a guiding principle of US and international child protection law. It considers factors such as a child's wishes, safety, and rights to development, family unity, liberty, and identity.[59] In a situation where a child's best interests are not guiding every policy decision, as is the case in our immigration system, policymakers will continue to put forward harmful policies. And where there are gaps in protection, as there are for both unaccompanied and accompanied children, the consequences will be dire.

In the absence of comprehensive policies and strategies to address the needs of children and their families fleeing violence in their countries of origin, local free clinics, federally qualified health centers, and community-based organizations are the best options for providing health care and support for these children and families. Undocumented and lawfully present immigrant children in the United States are at particularly high risk of lacking health insurance coverage; uninsurance rates are 33% for undocumented immigrant children and 18% for lawfully present immigrant children, compared with 4% for US citizen children with US-born citizen parents.[60] Nevertheless, only 6 states (CA, IL, MA, NY, OR, and WA) and Washington, DC, use state-only funds to cover income-eligible children, regardless of immigration status.[61] The substantial health-care and support needs of these vulnerable children and their families are best addressed by interdisciplinary teams consisting of pediatricians, social workers, counselors, psychologists and other behavioral health specialists, dentists, child advocacy specialists, certified interpreters, and immigration, refugee, and asylum attorneys. Although some practices may not have access to all members of such an interdisciplinary team, appropriate referrals should be made, especially to address the mental health-care needs and provide therapeutic interventions to mitigate the consequences of toxic stress, depression, anxiety, post-traumatic stress disorder, domestic violence, sexual assault, family separation, witnessing violence, and child abuse. Ideally, programs targeting the special needs of these vulnerable children and families should be supported by federal and state policies. In the absence of such policies and programs, clinicians can partner with local charitable organizations, community-based organizations, universities, and health systems to address the needs of these children and families.

Language barriers impact multiple aspects of health care, including access to care, health status, use of health services, patient–provider communication, satisfaction with care, quality of care, and patient safety.[62] Children and their families fleeing violence in their countries of origin frequently will confront language barriers in the United States owing to limited English proficiency. Such children and families should always be provided with trained professional medical interpreters and translators; not doing so actually violates Title VI federal mandates.[63] Ad hoc interpreters, such as children, family members, friends, and untrained staff, should never be used as interpreters or translators, given well-documented hazards that include significantly higher risks of committing interpretation errors of clinical consequence; avoidance of sensitive issues by family members when children interpret, such as domestic violence, drug use, and sexual assault; and patient-safety issues that can even include the death of siblings owing to misinterpretations.[53,64–66] A substantial number of children and families and from Mexico and Central and South America may speak an indigenous language as their primary language, and have limited or no fluency in Spanish or English. For example, 4.5 million people in Guatemala, Honduras, and El Salvador speak Mayan languages,[67] and 63 indigenous languages are spoken in Mexico, including Nahuatl by 1.4 million Mexicans.[68]

America's treatment of children and families fleeing violence is an issue of basic human compassion and human rights that speaks to the soul and morality of our country. Pediatricians have a substantial role to play in ensuring that policymakers heed their expertise on what is best for children's health, health care, development, and well-being. Pediatricians can raise awareness of and testify on how an administration's policies are intentionally cruel and harmful to children and families. Pediatricians can advocate for policies that protect the basic health and well-being of asylum-seeking children and families. **Table 1** lists legislation introduced by members of Congress that would protect immigrant children and their families. Pediatricians can be forceful

Table 1
Current federal bills under consideration that could benefit children and families forcibly displaced from their country of origin by violence

Bill Number	Bill Name	Sponsor	Date Introduced
H.R. 1012/S.557	REUNITE Act	Rep. Espaillat, Sen. Harris	2/6/19, 2/26/19
H.R. 3729/S. 661	Child Trafficking Victims Protection and Welfare Act	Rep. Roybal-Allard, Sen. Hirono	7/11/19, 3/5/19
S. 662	Fair Day in Court for Kids Act of 2019	Sen. Hirono	3/5/19
H.R. 2217	Families, Not Facilities Act of 2019	Rep. Wasserman Schultz	4/10/19
H.R. 2662	Asylum Seeker Protection Act	Rep. Escobar	5/10/19
S. 1733	Protecting Families and Improving Immigration Procedures Act	Sen. Feinstein	6/5/19
H.R. 3239/S. 2135	Humanitarian Standards for Individuals in Customs and Border Protection Custody Act	Rep. Ruiz, Sen. Udall	6/12/19, 7/17/19
H.R. 3451	Humane Enforcement and Legal Protections for Separated Children Act of 2019	Rep. Roybal-Allard	6/24/19
H.R. 3452	Help Separated Families Act of 2019	Rep. Roybal-Allard	6/24/19
H.R. 3918/S. 2113	Stop Cruelty to Migrant Children Act	Rep. Meng, Sen. Merkley	7/23/19, 7/15/19
S. 2256	Coordinating Care for Children Affected by Immigration Enforcement Act	Sen. Tina Smith	7/24/19
H.R. 5207	End the Migrant Protection Protocols Act of 2019	Rep. Vela	11/20/19
H.R. 5210/S. 2936	Refugee Protection Act of 2019	Rep. Lofgren, Sen. Leahy	11/21/19
H.R. 6437/S.3609	Coronavirus Immigrant Families Protection Act	Rep. Chu, Sen. Hirono	4/3/20, 5/5/20
H.R. 7569/S. 4011	Immigration Enforcement Moratorium Act	Rep. Wilson, Sen. Markey	7/9/20, 6/18/20

champions by calling their representatives, asking about their position on these bills, and advocating for legislators to cosponsor, consider, and pass them into law, as well as offering to provide testimony, writing op-eds, and leveraging blogs and social media.

SUMMARY

Children and their families in Mexico and Central and South America, as well as many children around the world, face multiple threats of violence, poverty, extortion, corruption, and increasing climate change in their communities. Seeking safety, health, and well-being for their children, many families flee to the United States. US immigration law and policy, however, has maintained prevention through deterrence policies, rather than shifting its asylum policy to protect children and families. The US government between 2016 and 2020, and at other times in our history, has implemented policies that have and will continue to harm children and families, making it more difficult for them to receive protection in the United States, and support once they are able to remain in the United States. Advocacy for a best-interest-of-the-child standards, evidence-based policies, and an interdisciplinary, multilingual team approach to health care will protect the safety, health, and well-being of immigrant children and families forcibly displaced from their home countries by violence.

CLINICS CARE POINTS

- Undocumented and lawfully present immigrant children in the US are at particularly high risk of lacking health-insurance coverage.

- The substantial healthcare and support needs of these vulnerable children and their families are best addressed by interdisciplinary teams consisting of pediatricians, social workers, counselors, psychologists and other behavioral-health specialists, dentists, child-advocacy specialists, certified interpreters, and immigration, refugee, and asylum attorneys.

- Children and their families fleeing violence in their countries of origin frequently will confront language barriers in the US due to limited English proficiency. Such children and families should always be provided with trained professional medical interpreters and translators.

DISCLOSURE

The authors have nothing to disclose.

REFERENCES

1. Children. UNHCR USA. Available at: https://www.unhcr.org/en-us/children-49c3646c1e8.html. Accessed November 6, 2020.
2. Figures at a Glance. UNHCR USA. 2020. Available at: https://www.unhcr.org/en-us/figures-at-a-glance.html. Accessed November 6, 2020.
3. Definitions: refugee, asylum seeker, IDP, migrant. HAIS. Available at: https://www.hias.org/sites/default/files/definitions_of_refugee2c_asylum_seeker2c_idp2c_and_migrant.pdf. Accessed November 6, 2020.
4. Sutton T, Restrepo D, Martinez J. Getting migration in the Americas Right. Center for American Progress. 2019. Available at: https://www.americanprogress.org/

issues/security/reports/2019/06/24/471322/getting-migration-americas-right/. Accessed September 4, 2020.

5. U.S. Border Patrol Southwest Border Apprehensions by Sector Fiscal Year 2020. U.S. Customs and Border Protection. Available at: https://www.cbp.gov/newsroom/stats/sw-border-migration/usbp-swborder-apprehensions. Accessed September 4, 2020.

6. Cheatham A. Central America's Turbulent Northern Triangle. Council on Foreign Relations. 2019. Available at: https://www.cfr.org/backgrounder/central-americas-turbulent-northern-triangle. Accessed September 4, 2020.

7. Homicide Mortality by State. Centers for Disease Control and Prevention. 2020. Available at: https://www.cdc.gov/nchs/pressroom/sosmap/homicide_mortality/homicide.htm. Accessed November 6, 2020.

8. Beittel JS. Mexico: organized crime and drug trafficking organizations. Congressional Research Service; 2020. Available at: https://fas.org/sgp/crs/row/R41576.pdf. Accessed September 3, 2020.

9. Economic Commission for Latin America and the Caribbean. ECLAC: at least 2,795 women were victims of femicide in 23 Countries of Latin America and the Caribbean in 2017. Economic Commission for Latin America and the Caribbean. 2018. Available at: https://www.cepal.org/en/pressreleases/eclac-least-2795-women-were-victims-femicide-23-countries-latin-america-and-caribbean. Accessed September 4, 2020.

10. Sandin L. Femicides in Mexico: impunity and protests. Center for Strategic and International Studies; 2020. Available at: https://www.csis.org/analysis/femicides-mexico-impunity-and-protests. Accessed September 4, 2020.

11. Economic Commission for Latin America and the Caribbean (ECLAC). Poverty in Latin America: one of the critical obstacles to sustainable development. Social Panorama of Latin America 2019. Santiago (Chile): United Nations; 2019. p. 89–118. Available at: https://repositorio.cepal.org/bitstream/handle/11362/44989/1/S1901132_en.pdf. Accessed January 7, 2021.

12. 2019 Corruption Perceptions Index. Transparency International. 2020. Available at: https://www.transparency.org/en/cpi. Accessed September 4, 2020.

13. Project TCR. How is climate change affecting Mexico? The Climate Reality Project. 2018. Available at: https://www.climaterealityproject.org/blog/how-climate-change-affecting-mexico. Accessed September 4, 2020.

14. Aldrich J, Arvey S, Lopez G. The release of families seeking asylum across the U.S. Southwest border. University of California, San Diego School of Global Policy and Strategy; 2009. Available at: https://ccis.ucsd.edu/_files/Publications/QuickReleaseReport.pdf. Accessed September 3, 2020.

15. UN General Assembly, Convention Relating to the Status of Refugees, 28 July 1951. Available at: https://www.refworld.org/docid/3be01b964.html. Accessed 11 September 2020.

16. Asylum in the United States. American Immigration Council. 2020. Available at: https://www.americanimmigrationcouncil.org/research/asylum-united-states. Accessed September 3, 2020. (13).

17. National Standards on Transports, Escort, Detention, and Search. Section 4.1 U.S. Customs and Border Protection. 2015. Available at: https://www.cbp.gov/sites/default/files/assets/documents/2020-Feb/cbp-teds-policyoctober2015.pdf. Accessed September 3, 2020.

18. Cantor G. Detained beyond the limit: prolonged confinement by U.S. customs and border protection along the Southwest border. American Immigration Council; 2016. Available at: https://www.americanimmigrationcouncil.org/research/

prolongeddetention-us-customs-border-protection. Accessed September 3, 2020.

19. Family Detention. Detention Watch Network. Available at: https://www. detentionwatchnetwork.org/issues/family-detention. Accessed September 4, 2020.

20. 8 U.S.C. § 1158(b)(1)(B)(i).

21. Brown A, Wheeler C. Immigrating the Spouse and Children of Refugees Asylees. United States Conference of Catholic Bishops. Available at: https://www.usccb.org/ offices/children-andmigration/immigrating-spouse-and-children-refugees-asylees. Accessed September 4, 2020.

22. Green Card for Asylees. USCIS. Available at: https://www.uscis.gov/green-card/ green-cardeligibility/green-card-forasylees#:~:text=U.S.%20immigration%20law %20allows%20asylees,(get%20a%20Green%20Card). Accessed September 4, 2020.

23. Broder T, Moussavain A, Blazer J. Overview of immigrant eligibility for federal pro-grams. National Immigration Law Center; 2015. Available at: https://www.nilc.org/ issues/economic-support/overview-immeligfedprograms. Accessed September 4, 2020.

24. 6 U.S.C. § 279(g).

25. 8 U.S.C. § 1232.

26. Stipulated Settlement Agreement, Flores v. Reno, No.CV 85-4544-RJK (Px) (C.D. Cal. Jan. 17, 1997).

27. Kao K, Lu D. How Trump's Policies Are Leaving Thousands of Asylum Seekers Wait-ing in Mexico. New York Times. 2019. Available at: https://www.nytimes.com/ interactive/2019/08/18/us/mexico-immigration-asylum.html. Accessed September 3, 2020.

28. Trump Administration Sending Asylum Seekers and Migrants to Danger. Human Rights First. Available at: https://www.humanrightsfirst.org/campaign/remain-mexico. Accessed September 3, 2020.

29. U.S. Immigration Policy on Haitian Migrants. Congressional Research Service. 2011. Available at: https://www.everycrsreport.com/files/20110517_RS21349_ c6a8bc391c450f3244b0151c20deab7110d31290.pdf. Accessed November 6, 2020.

30. Alvarez P. 'I don't want to be deported': inside the tent courts on the US-Mexico border. CNN; 2020. Available at: https://www.cnn.com/2020/01/28/politics/tent-courts-remain-in-mexico/index.html. Accessed September 3, 2020.

31. Alvarez P. At least 350 children of migrant families forced to remain in Mexico have crossed over alone to US. CNN; 2020. Available at: https://www.cnn.com/2020/01/ 24/politics/migrant-children-remain-in-mexico/index.html. Accessed September 3, 2020.

32. Dickerson C. 'There is a Stench': soiled clothes and no baths for migrant children at a Texas Center. New York Times 2019. Available at: https://www.nytimes.com/ 2019/06/21/us/migrant-children-border-soap.html. Accessed September 3, 2020.

33. Fink S, Dickerson C. Border patrol facilities put detainees with medical conditions at risk. 2019. Available at: https://www.nytimes.com/2019/03/05/us/border-patrol-deaths-migrant-children.html. Accessed September 11, 2020.

34. Hennessy-Fiske M. Six migrant children have died in U.S. custody. Here's what we know about them. 2019. Available at: https://www.latimes.com/nation/lana-migrant-child-border-deaths-20190524-story.html. Accessed September 3, 2020.

35. Trump Administration's Third Country Transit Bar is an asylum ban that will return refugees to danger. Human Rights First. 2019. Available at: https://www.

humanrightsfirst.org/sites/default/files/Third-Country-Transit-Ban.pdf. Accessed September 4, 2020.

36. Reichlin-Melnick A. What you need to know about Trump's proposal to eliminate the US Asylum System. Immigration Impact. 2020. Available at: https://immigrationimpact.com/2020/06/11/end-asylum-trump/#.X1JSZ2dKjlw. Accessed September 4, 2020.

37. Pandemic as pretext: Trump administration exploits COVID-19, expels asylum seekers and children's to escalating danger. Human Rights First. 2020. Available at: https://www.humanrightsfirst.org/sites/default/files/PandemicAsPretextFINAL.pdf. Accessed September 4, 2020.

38. Nationwide enforcement encounters: Title 8 enforcement action and title 42 expulsions. U.S. Customs and Border Protection. Available at: https://www.cbp.gov/newsroom/stats/cbp-enforcementstatistics/title-8-and-title-42-statistics. Accessed September 4, 2020.

39. Merchant N. AP exclusive: migrant kids held in US hotels, then expelled. AP. 2020. Available at: https://apnews.com/c9b671b206060f2e9654f0a4eaeb6388. Accessed September 4, 2020.

40. Public Health Experts Urge U.S. Officials to Withdraw Order Enabling Mass Expulsion of Asylum Seekers. Columbia Mailman School of Public Health. 2020. Available at: https://www.publichealth.columbia.edu/public-health-now/news/public-health-experts-urge-us-officials-withdraw-order-enabling-mass-exp ulsion-asylum-seekers. Accessed September 11, 2020.

41. Public Health Measures to Safely Manage Asylum Seekers and Children at the Border. Human Rights First. 2020. Available at: https://www.humanrightsfirst.org/sites/default/files/PublicHealthMeasuresattheBorder.05.18.2020.pdf. Accessed September 11, 2020.

42. The Family Case Management Program: why case management can and must be part of the US approach to immigration. Women's Refugee Commission. 2019. Available at: https://s33660 pcdn.co/wp-content/uploads/2020/04/The-Family-Case-Management-Program.pdf. Accessed September 11, 2020.

43. Aguilera J. 120 children remain in ICE detention despite court order for them to be released due to COVID-19 concerns. Time. 2020. Available at: https://time.com/5878909/children-ice-covid-19-detention-court-order/. Accessed September 4, 2020.

44. Lutheran Immigration and Refugee Service, The Women's Refugee Commission. Locking up family values, again. Baltimore (MD): Lutheran Immigration and Refugee Service; 2014. Available at: https://www.lirs.org/assets/2474/lirswrc_lockingupfamilyvaluesagain_report_141114.pdf. Accessed September 8, 2020.

45. Flores v. Lynch, Case No. 2:85-cv-04544-DMG-AGR. February 23, 2016. Available at: https://www.humanrightsfirst.org/sites/default/files/HRFFloresAmicusBrief.pdf. Accessed September 8, 2020.

46. Linton JM, Griffin M, Shapiro AJ, et al, AAP Council on Community Pediatrics. Detention of immigrant children. Pediatrics 2017;139(5):e20170483.

47. Eagly I, Shafer S, Whalley J. Detaining families: a study of asylum adjudication in family detention. American Immigration Council; 2018. Available at: https://www.americanimmigrationcouncil.org/sites/default/files/research/detaining_families_a_st udy_of_asylum_adjudication_in_family_detention_final.pdf. Accessed September 11, 2020.

48. Seville LR, Rappleye H. Trump admin ran 'pilot program' for separating migrant families in 2017. NBC News 2018. Available at: https://www.nbcnews.com/

storyline/immigration-border-crisis/trump-admin-ran-pilot-programseparating-migrant-families-2017-n887616. Accessed September 3, 2020.

49. Spagat E. Tally of children split at border tops 5,400 in new count. AP News 2019. Available at: https://apnews.com/c654e652a4674cf19304a4a4ff599feb. Accessed September 3, 2020.

50. Family separation is not over: how the Trump administration continues to separate children from their parents to serve its political ends. Young Center for Immigrant Children's Rights. 2020. Available at: https://static1.squarespace.com/static/597ab5f3bebafb0a625aaf45/t/5f032e87ff32c80f99c7fee5/1594044048699/Young+Center-Family+Separation+Report-Final+PDF.pdf. Accessed September 3, 2020.

51. Ainsley J, Soboroff J. Lawyers say they can't find parents of 545 migrant children separated by Trump administration. 2020. Available at: https://www.nbcnews.com/politics/immigration/lawyers-say-they-can-t-find-parents-545-migrant-children-n1244066. Accessed November 6, 2020.

52. Physicians for Human Rights. "You will never see your child again": the persistent psychological effects of family separation. 2020. Available at: https://phr.org/wp-content/uploads/2020/02/PHR-Report-2020-Family-Separation-Full-Report.pdf. Accessed September 11, 2020.

53. Capps R, Koball H, Campetella A, et al. Implications of immigration enforcement activities for the well-being of children in immigrant families. Urban Institute, Migration Policy Institute; 2015. Available at: https://www.urban.org/sites/default/files/alfresco/publication-exhibits/2000405/2000405-Implications-of-Immigration-Enforcement-Activities-for-the-Well-Being-of-Children-in-Immigrant-Families.pdf. Accessed September 10, 2020.

54. FAQs on changes to the employment authorization rules for asylum seekers. CLINIC. 2020. Available at: https://cliniclegal.org/resources/removal-proceedings/defensiveasylum/faqs-changes-employment-authorization-rules-asylum. Accessed September 4, 2020.

55. Changes to public charge: analysis and frequently asked questions. Protecting Immigrant Families. 2020. Available at: https://docs.google.com/document/d/1zHLRaciDqIZfkl_icRGVJWKWcinP6cAwvkuAeae8eog/edit. Accessed September 4, 2020.

56. Trump's public charge regulation is hurting immigrant families now. Protecting Immigrant Families. 2020. Available at: https://protectingimmigrantfamilies.org/wpcontent/uploads/2020/04/DocumentingHarm-update-2020-04-27.pdf. Accessed September 4, 2020.

57. Perreira KM, Pedroza JM. Policies of exclusion: implications for the health of immigrants and their children. Annu Rev Public Health 2019;40:147–66.

58. Christi M, Bolter J. Vulnerable to COVID-19 in frontline jobs, immigrants are mostly shut out of U.S. relief. Migration Policy Institute. 2020. Available at: https://www.migrationpolicy.org/article/covid19-immigrants-shut-out-federalrelief. Accessed September 4, 2020.

59. Framework for Considering the Best Interests of Unaccompanied Children. Subcommittee on Best Interests of the Interagency Working Group on Unaccompanied and Separated Children. 2016. Available at: https://static1.squarespace.com/static/597ab5f3bebafb0a625aaf45/t/5c19cb386d2a738d43742361/1545194298896/Best-Interests-Framework.pdf. Accessed September 10, 2020.

60. Kaiser Family Foundation. Health coverage of immigrants. 2020. Available at: https://www.kff.org/racial-equity-and-health-policy/fact-sheet/health-coverage-of-immigrants/. Accessed September 15, 2020.

61. Artiga S, Diaz M. Health coverage and care of undocumented immigrants. Kaiser Family Foundation; 2019. Available at: https://www.kff.org/racial-equity-and-health-policy/issue-brief/health-coverage-and-care-of-undocumented-immigrants/. Accessed September 15, 2020.

62. Flores G. The impact of medical interpreter services on the quality of health care: a systematic review. Med Care Res Rev 2005;62(3):255–99. https://doi.org/10.1177/1077558705275416.

63. Hayashi D. Guidance memorandum. Title VI prohibition against national origin discrimination—persons with limited English proficiency. Washington, DC: U.S. Department of Health & Human Services; 1998.

64. Flores G, Laws MB, Mayo SJ, et al. Errors in medical interpretation and their potential clinical consequences in pediatric encounters. Pediatrics 2003;111(1): 6–14. https://doi.org/10.1542/peds.111.1.6.

65. Flores G. Families facing language barriers in healthcare: when will policy catch up with the demographics and evidence? J Pediatr 2014;164(6):1261–4.

66. Mosquera RA, Samuels C, Flores G. Family language barriers and special-needs children. Pediatrics 2016;138(4):e20160321.

67. Native Languages of the Americas. Most Common Central American Languages (by number of speakers today). Available at: http://www.native-languages.org/most-central.htm. Accessed September 15, 2020.

68. Čirjak A. How Many Native Languages Are Spoken In Mexico? World Atlas. 2020. Available at: https://www.worldatlas.com/how-many-native-languages-are-spoken-in-mexico.html. Accessed September 15, 2020.

An Eye on Disparities, Health Equity, and Racism— The Case of Firearm Injuries in Urban Youth in the United States and Globally

Margaret K. Formica, MSPH, PhD

KEYWORDS

- Firearm violence • Youth • Urban • Disparities • Health equity • Racism
- Epidemiology

KEY POINTS

- Firearm violence is a significant public health problem, particularly among children and adolescents in the United States.
- Racial disparities in firearm violence among urban youth exists, disproportionately affecting Black men.
- Evidence of the role of racism in the disparate rates of firearm violence among urban Black men is presented.
- Firearm violence prevention efforts targeted at social determinants of health, including racism, are needed to achieve health equity.

The morning of Saturday June 20th, 2020, 17-year-old Chariel Osoria attended his graduation from Corcoran High School in Syracuse, NY. After spending time at a small graduation party in his honor at his mother's house, he stopped by "Rye Day" party— an annual outdoor event held for the last 14 years. It is unclear how the event was held given the restrictions in place due to the COVID-19 pandemic, but there were several hundred people at the party. As the event was winding down early in the evening, several gunshots rang out—by the time the dust settled 9 people were injured, including Chariel, who was shot in the head.[1]

NATURE OF THE PROBLEM

Unfortunately, the story of Chariel is not unique. In 2018, almost 40,000 people died as a result of firearm injuries in the United States.[2] With more than twice as many nonfatal

Department of Public Health and Preventive Medicine, State University of New York Upstate Medical University, 750 East Adams Street, Syracuse, NY 13210, USA
E-mail address: formicam@upstate.edu

Pediatr Clin N Am 68 (2021) 389–399
https://doi.org/10.1016/j.pcl.2020.12.009   pediatric.theclinics.com
0031-3955/21/© 2020 Elsevier Inc. All rights reserved.

firearm injuries as fatal injuries,[3] well more than 300 people are injured or killed by fire-arms in the United States every day.

Most other countries do not contend with the same level of firearm violence as the United States. Two recent studies comparing firearm mortality across countries indi-cate that a high proportion of global firearm violence is occurring in the United States.[4,5] The United States, ranking second in total firearm deaths, is 1 of 6 countries (which also includes Brazil, Colombia, Guatemala, Mexico, and Venezuela) that contribute to more than half of all firearm deaths worldwide, despite reflecting less than 10% of the global population.[5] Furthermore, when the United States is compared with only other high-income countries, the firearm death rate is 11.4 times higher.[4]

Chariel is part of an age group that is particularly burdened by firearm violence. Among adolescents and young adults aged 15 to 24 years in the United States, suicide and homicide are the second and third leading causes of death, respectively,[6] and firearms are responsible for most of those deaths.[7] In fact, when we focus on children and adolescents aged 1 to 19 years, firearm injuries result in 15% of all deaths, are the second leading cause of death in that age group, and have been increasing since 2013.[8] And again, the United States is outpacing most of the world in firearm violence among adolescents and young adults. Based on data from the 2017 Global Burden of Disease Study, the incidence of physical violence by firearm among youth aged 15 to 24 years indicates that the US rate is second only to Venezuela and substantially higher than most other countries (**Fig. 1**). Firearm violence is clearly a significant public health problem, particularly among children and adolescents in the United States.

Rates of firearm violence are often described according to the type—homicide/as-sault, suicide/self-harm, and unintentional—and although in the United States the overall rate of suicide by firearm is more than twice that of homicide,[4] the opposite

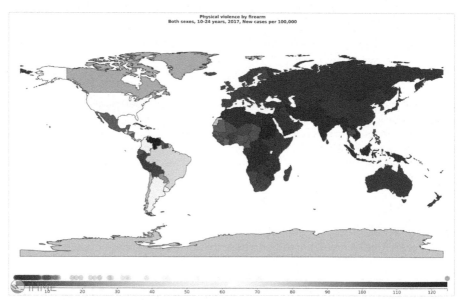

Fig. 1. Global map of the incidence of physical violence by firearm per 100,000 among those aged 10 to 24 years by country, 2017 Global Burden of Disease Study. Institute for Health Metrics and Evaluation (IHME). GBD Compare Data Visualization. Seattle, WA: IHME, University of Washington. Available from http://vizhub.healthdata.org/gbd-compare. (Accessed July 19, 2020).

is true for children and adolescents. Among those aged 1 to 19 years, almost 60% of firearm fatalities are homicides, 35% are suicides, and the remaining are unintentional or undetermined.[8] There is also variability in the type of firearm violence among youth—unintentional firearm injuries are more common among younger children, whereas homicide and suicide are more common among adolescents.[9]

In addition to variations in types of firearm violence by age, there are also substantial urban/rural differences. In 2017, overall death rates from firearm injuries among youth were similar in rural and urban communities (4.45 vs 4.29 per 100,000). However, although youth from rural areas were more likely to die from self-inflicted and unintentional firearm injuries, urban youth were more than 2 times as likely to die from firearm homicide.[8] Recent research on firearm injury hospitalizations in children and adolescents further supports the urban/rural divide, as well as highlights the crisis among urban adolescents aged 15 to 19 years. Findings from Herrin and colleagues (2018) indicate that by far, the highest rates of hospitalizations for firearm injuries are among those 15 to 19 years of age, particularly from urban areas (30.7 per 100,000). And, when focused in on the age group of 15 to 19 years, the high firearm injury hospitalization rate among those from urban communities is driven, primarily by assaults, reflecting 70% of those hospitalizations.[10]

DISPARITIES IN URBAN FIREARM VIOLENCE

Although firearm violence is the leading cause of death and injury among urban youth, a closer look indicates there are substantial disparities with respect to gender and race. Regardless of the data source or setting, young Black men have consistently been found to be disproportionately affected by firearm injuries and deaths.[8–17] At the national level for example, Fowler and colleagues[13] (2016) found that non-Hispanic Black youth aged 15 to 24 years were 19 times as likely to be victims of firearm homicide than their non-Hispanic White peers. More recent data demonstrate the same disparity, as well as the contrast between metro and nonmetro areas. Using data from National Fatal Injury Reports from 2018, firearm homicide death rates among those aged 15 to 24 years were substantially higher for non-Hispanic Black men compared with Non-Hispanic White men, with the largest disparity for those living in metro areas (**Fig. 2**).[3]

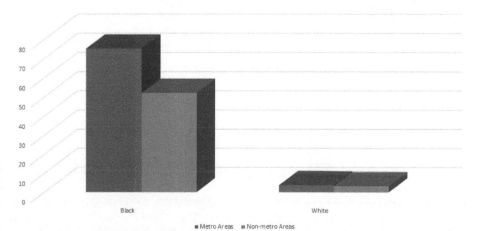

Fig. 2. US Firearm homicide deaths per 100,000 among men aged 15 to 24 years by race, National Fatal Injury Reports, 2018.

Research within urban centers has identified similar patterns.[11,18] One such study using police data in Philadelphia found that 82% of firearm assault victims were Black and 92% were men.[11] The city of Syracuse, NY, where Chariel and 8 others were shot at the "Rye Day" party experiences similar patterns of firearm violence. Utilizing previously unpublished data from the Syracuse City Police Department between 2010 and 2016 and Census Bureau population estimates, the rates of shots fired per 100,000 (including both injury and homicide) were the highest among younger age groups, and 12 times higher for both men compared with women (112.5 vs 9.4) and Black compared with White victims (167.2 vs 13.9) (**Fig. 3**A–C).

A focus on death and injury statistics alone does not adequately address the extent of the burden of firearm violence. The economic loss associated with firearm violence is striking. Based on average annual firearm injuries and deaths between 2010 and 2012, the total lifetime costs of firearm injuries and deaths from work loss and medical costs is greater than $48 billion, and firearm assaults alone are greater than $20 billion.[13] Economic burden aside, there are also long-term physical and behavioral consequences that can be attributed to victimization and witnessing firearm violence among youth. And just as Black youth are more likely to be victims of firearm injuries and deaths in urban settings, they are also more likely to be witness to it.[19] A recent scoping review of the long-term consequences of youth exposure to firearm injury found strong evidence of associations with posttraumatic stress disorder and increased likelihood of future firearm injury.[20] In addition, youth exposure to firearm violence contributes to adverse childhood experiences, which have been linked to physical and psychological conditions, increased risk behaviors, developmental disruption, and health care utilization.[21]

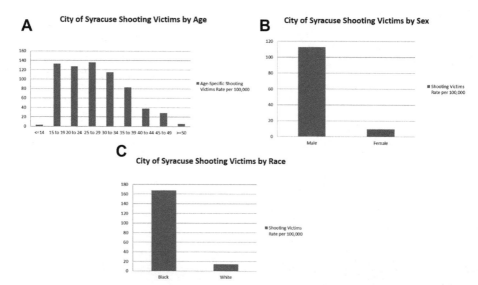

Fig. 3. (A) Shootings resulting in injury or homicide in the City of Syracuse per 100,000 by age group, Syracuse City Police Department data, 2010 to 2016. (B) Shootings resulting in injury or homicide in the City of Syracuse per 100,000 by sex, Syracuse City Police Department data, 2010 to 2016. (C) Shootings resulting in injury or homicide in the City of Syracuse per 100,000 by race, Syracuse City Police Department data, 2010 to 2016.

CURRENT EVIDENCE

So, what is driving these disparities in urban firearm violence? Arguably, the most well-established community-level predictor of crime is poverty.[22–25] The indicators of concentrated disadvantage, including poverty, have been described as the "strongest and most stable" predictors of crime, including firearm violence, in a meta-analysis.[24] For example, among youth aged 15 to 24 years in California, 81% of homicides occurred in neighborhoods with poverty levels of 20% or greater, whereas only 2% or homicides occurred in neighborhoods with low levels of poverty.[23]

The city where Chariel was shot, Syracuse, is a midsized city in Central New York with a population of 145,170 in 2010.[26] The city is considered one of the most impoverished in the country, with one-third of all residents living below the federal poverty level,[26] and in 2015 was ranked first in the nation in concentrated poverty among Blacks and Hispanics.[27] In 2013, the per capita murder rate in Syracuse topped all cities in New York State.[28] Comprehensive information on firearm violence for the city of Syracuse is sparse, although crime-related shooting statistics indicate that the city is disproportionately affected by gun violence.[29] The Syracuse Police Department data on shootings from 2010 to 2016 described earlier indicate an annual age-adjusted homicide rate of 6.1 per 100,000, which is almost 1.7 times the national rate.[30] And, the economic impact of gun violence on the city has been extensive—a study using data from 2006 to 2008 calculated that just the emergency medical care for each gunshot victim totaled $28,510,[31] with much greater costs for the continuing care of those injured. Multiplying that estimated cost of emergency care to treat each gunshot victim by the number of such injuries in Syracuse suggests that Medicaid costs simply to cover the emergency care of gunshot injuries was greater than $2.5 million per year.

Geospatial analysis of the Syracuse City Police Department data on rates of firearm injury and homicide supports the association between neighborhood concentrated poverty and firearm violence (**Fig. 4**). Poverty at the census block level was determined using Census data of the proportion of the population living below poverty level.[26] In general, census blocks with the highest rate of firearm assaults align with those that have the highest proportion of the population living in poverty. However, not all impoverished Syracuse neighborhoods are affected by firearm violence uniformly; some census blocks with higher poverty levels experienced relatively low levels of firearm violence and vice-versa, indicating other factors may be playing a role.

Recent research examining the relationship between firearm violence and neighborhood income have found that both firearm homicides and hospitalizations are linked to economic disadvantage,[11,12,32] although the relationship may be more complex than initially understood. When compared with pedestrian motor vehicle hospitalizations, children from poor neighborhoods were at greater risk of firearm hospitalizations; however, for Black children the increased risk was not attenuated by living in a more affluent neighborhood.[12] Further exploring these relationships, Beard and colleagues[11] (2017) found that Black residents of Philadelphia experienced the same degree of firearm assaults regardless of income and hypothesized that other structural circumstances, such as racial segregation, may be factors in the increased risk of firearm violence. Public health research building on this theory has shown that racial segregation does likely increase the firearm homicide disparities between Black and White populations,[33,34] as does income inequality.[32,35,36]

ROLE OF RACISM

Racial segregation in the United States is rooted in a long history of structural racism. Structural racism can be considered as, "the processes of racism that are embedded

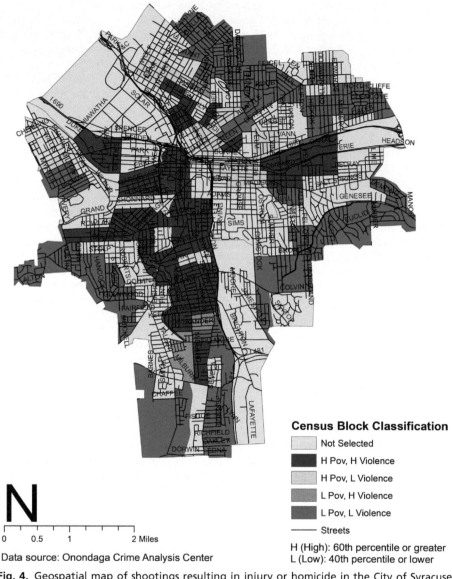

**Syracuse Block Groups Classified by Poverty Rates and
Mean Annual Rate of Gunshot Injuries and Homicides
Syracuse, NY, Jan. 1, 2010 - Mar. 23, 2016**

Census Block Classification

- Not Selected
- H Pov, H Violence
- H Pov, L Violence
- L Pov, H Violence
- L Pov, L Violence
- —— Streets

H (High): 60th percentile or greater
L (Low): 40th percentile or lower

Data source: Onondaga Crime Analysis Center

Fig. 4. Geospatial map of shootings resulting in injury or homicide in the City of Syracuse per 100,000 and poverty level.

in laws (local, state, and federal), policies, and practices of society and its institutions that provide advantages to racial groups deemed as superior, while differentially oppressing, disadvantaging, or otherwise neglecting other racial groups viewed as inferior".[37] As so eloquently described in their paper on structural racism and health inequities, Bailey and colleagues[38] (2017) summarize a history of structural racism in the United States. With examples from the legalization of slavery, subsequent Jim

Crow legislation, the exclusion of occupations predominantly held by Black workers from the 1935 Social Security Act, to private sector racially discriminatory policies and practices on employment, housing, etc., the paper distinctly conveys the multi-generational disadvantages that have led to ongoing racial segregation.

One example of structural racism that has received a good detail of media attention, as well as attention in the public health literature as it relates to health disparities, is "redlining." In the 1930s, the Home Owners' Loan Corporation was commissioned to create maps of 239 cities in the United States and rate neighborhoods within each city based on the security of the investment. Neighborhoods deemed the highest risk, predominantly minority neighborhoods, were marked in red, and private lenders subsequently used these maps to engage in discriminatory lending practices, perpetuating urban segregation and concentrated poverty.[39,40] Racial disparities for a wide range of health outcomes from self-reported general health, asthma, myocardial infarction, and maternal and child health outcomes to cancer diagnoses and survival have all been linked to redlining.[41–46]

There is also a growing body of research specifically around the association between the practice of redlining and violence, including rates of firearm-related injuries and deaths. In a spatial analysis of firearm assaults and violent crime in 2013 to 2014 and redlining in Philadelphia, Jacoby and colleagues (2018) found the highest rates in the neighborhoods that were historically redlined.[11] In similar research in Louisville, KY, gunshot victims between 2012 and 2018 were more likely to be from historically redlined communities.[40] This research has critically called attention to the role of historical and ongoing structural racism that has led to the existing disproportionate burden of firearm violence that young, urban Black men face in the United States.

Structural racism is likely a key contributing factor to the high rates of urban firearm violence experienced by Black youth, but cultural racism biases how it is perceived in American society. Cultural racism is "the instillation of the ideology of inferiority in the values, language, imagery, symbols and unstated assumptions of the larger society."[37] The media often frames gun-related crime among minorities, and particularly, low-income minorities, as an individual problem with at least some degree of blame placed on the victims. Gun-related crime among nonminorities, on the other hand, is more likely to be framed as a shared problem with innocent victims.[47] Consequently, urban gun violence, which disproportionately affects Black men receives very little attention from a societal and political standpoint.

Even the dialogue around urban gun violence as compared with other public health problems that primarily affect Whites is reflective of cultural racism. For several years, there has been growing interest and research in "deaths of despair"—drug poisonings, suicides, and diseases related to alcoholism[48]—a phrase conceived in a 2015 paper that discussed the increase in mortality from those diseases among middle-aged non-Hispanic Whites.[49] A follow-up to that paper further described "deaths of despair" as resulting from cumulative disadvantage.[50] Despair, or loss of hope, provides the connotation of minimizing individual responsibility in favor of societal responsibility. Interestingly, the cumulative disadvantage suffered by generations of Blacks has not warranted the inclusion of urban firearm violence in the list of "deaths of despair." In contrast, urban gun violence is often described as a disease of poverty securing the perception of individual responsibility.

CURRENT COMPLICATIONS

The COVID-19 pandemic, and to some extent, the social unrest following the murder of George Floyd have brought racial health disparities into the national discourse.

Ironically, the very issues that exposed the problem may increase firearm violence and its disparities. A yet-to-be-published study conducted by researchers at University of California Davis and the University of California Firearm Violence Research Center found that between March and May of 2020, an excess of an estimated 2.1 million firearms were sold and during that same time period, the United States saw a corresponding 8% increase in firearm violence.[51] In addition, the economic devastation caused by COVID-19 has disproportionately affected minority populations, potentially exacerbating the conditions that lead to violence.[52]

RECOMMENDATIONS

On June 25th 2020, Chariel died from the firearm injuries he sustained 5 days earlier at the "Rye Day" party. It has been reported that he was trying to deescalate a disagreement between members of rival gangs when the shooting began. Chariel was a new high school graduate with hopes, dreams, and plans for his future, all cut short by firearm violence that was preventable. Although prevention efforts are a focus of other articles in this issue, it is clear that racial disparities do exist with respect to firearm violence, and prevention needs to be considered within that context. To minimize deaths and injuries due to firearms and their cascading health consequences, particularly in urban settings, and to ultimately achieve health equity, preventive efforts will need to address the social determinants of health, including racism.

CLINICAL CARE POINTS

- Firearm violence is a leading cause of death among adolescents and young adults in the United States.
- Unintentional firearm injuries are more common among young children, whereas homicide and suicide by firearm are more common among adolescents.
- Long-term physical and behavioral consequences among youth can be attributed to victimization and witness of firearm violence.
- Young Black men in urban settings are disproportionately affected by firearm injuries and deaths.
- Poverty and racism are key contributing factors to the high rates of urban firearm violence experienced by Black youth.
- The COVID-19 pandemic is potentially exacerbating the conditions that lead to firearm violence.

DISCLOSURE

The author has nothing to disclose.

ACKNOWLEDGEMENT

The author would like to acknowledge and thank Donald Cibula for his time and expertise in the creation of the geospatial map of shootings resulting in injury or homicide and poverty level in Syracuse (**Figure 4**).

REFERENCES

1. Dowty D. Syracuse teen shot at party graduated 6 hours before; family says he's not expected to survive. The post-standard. Available at: https://www.syracuse.

com/crime/2020/06/syracuse-teen-mortally-wounded-in-mass-party-shooting-had-graduated-high-school-6-hours-before.html. Accessed August 4, 2020.

2. Centers for Disease Control and Prevention (CDC). Web-based injury statistics query and reporting systems: Fatal injury data visualization explore. Available at: https://wisqars-viz.cdc.gov:8006/explore-data/home. Accessed July 25, 2020.

3. Centers for Disease Control and Prevention (CDC). Web-based injury statistics query and reporting systems: Nonfatal injury reports. Available at: https://webappa.cdc.gov/sasweb/ncipc/nfirates.html. Accessed July 25, 2020.

4. Grinshteyn E, Hemenway D. Violent death rates: The US Compared with other high-income OECD Countries, 2010. Am J Med 2016;129(3):266–73.

5. Global Burden of Disease 2016 Injury Collaborators. Global mortality from firearms, 1990-2016. J Am Med Assoc 2018;320(8):792–814.

6. Centers for Disease Control and Prevention (CDC). Web-based injury statistics query and reporting systems: leading causes of death reports. Available at: https://webappa.cdc.gov/sasweb/ncipc/leadcause.html. Accessed July 25, 2020.

7. Anglemyer A, Horvath T, Rutherford G. The accessibility of firearms and risk for suicide and homicide victimization among household members a systematic review and meta-analysis. Ann Intern Med 2014;160(2):101–10. Available at: www.annals.org.

8. Cunningham RM, Walton MA, Carter PM. The major causes of death in children and adolescents in the United States. N Engl J Med 2018;379:2468–75.

9. Fowler KA, Dahlberg LL, Haileyesus T, et al. Childhood firearm injuries in the United States. Pediatrics 2017;140(1):e20163486.

10. Herrin BR, Gaither JR, Leventhal JM, et al. Rural versus urban hospitalizations for firearm injuries in children and adolescents. Pediatrics 2018;142(2):e20173318.

11. Beard JH, Morrison CN, Jacoby SF, et al. Quantifying disparities in urban firearm violence by race and place in Philadelphia, Pennsylvania: a cartographic study. Am J Public Health 2017;107(3):371–3.

12. Kalesan B, Vyliparambil MA, Bogue E, et al. Race and ethnicity, neighborhood poverty and pediatric firearm hospitalizations in the United States. Ann Epidemiol 2016;26(1):1–6.e2.

13. Fowler KA, Dahlberg LL, Haileyesus T, et al. Firearm injuries in the United States. Prev Med (Baltim) 2015;79:5–14.

14. Martin CA, Unni P, Landman MP, et al. Race disparities in firearm injuries and outcomes among Tennessee children. J Pediatr Surg 2012;47:1196–203. W.B. Saunders.

15. Pressley JC, Barlow B, Kendig T, et al. Twenty-year trends in fatal injuries to very young children: the persistence of racial disparities. Pediatrics 2007;119(4). https://doi.org/10.1542/peds.2006-2412.

16. Leventhal JM, Gaither JR, Sege R. Hospitalizations due to firearm injuries in children and adolescents. Pediatrics 2014;133(2):219–25.

17. Srinivasan S, Mannix R, Lee LK. Epidemiology of paediatric firearm injuries in the USA, 2001-2010. Arch Dis Child 2014;99(4):331–5.

18. Walker GN, McLone S, Mason M, et al. Rates of firearm homicide by Chicago region, age, sex, and race/ethnicity, 2005-2010. J Trauma Acute Care Surg 2016. https://doi.org/10.1097/TA.0000000000001176.

19. Fowler PJ, Tompsett CJ, Braciszewski JM, et al. Community violence: a meta-analysis on the effect of exposure and mental health outcomes of children and adolescents. Dev Psychopathol 2009. https://doi.org/10.1017/S0954579409000145.

20. Ranney M, Karb R, Ehrlich P, et al. What are the long-term consequences of youth exposure to firearm injury, and how do we prevent them? A scoping review. J Behav Med 2019;42(4):724–40.

21. Kalmakis KA, Chandler GE. Health consequences of adverse childhood experiences: a systematic review. J Am Assoc Nurse Pract 2015;27(8):457–65.

22. Sampson RJ, Raudenbush SW, Earls F. Neighborhoods and violent crime: a multilevel study of collective efficacy. Science 1997;277(5328):918–24.

23. Males M. Age, poverty, homicide, and gun homicide: is young age or poverty level the key issue? SAGE Open Med 2015;5(1). 2158244015573359.

24. Pratt TC, Cullen FT. Assessing macro-level predictors and theories of crime: a meta-analysis. Crime Justice 2005;32:373–450.

25. Sampson R. Great American city: Chicago and the enduring neighborhood effect. Chicago (IL): University of Chicago Press; 2012.

26. United States Census Bureau (Census). American FactFinder. Available at: http://factfinder.census.gov/faces/nav/jsf/pages/index.xhtml. Accessed April 16, 2016.

27. Jargowsky P. The architecture of segregation: civil unrest, the concentration of poverty, and public policy. The Century foundation. Available at: http://apps.tcf.org/architecture-of-segregation. Accessed April 18, 2016.

28. Dowty D, Stein J. Syracuse's 15 homicides more than last year; if pace continues, 2013 will be the worst year in city's history. The Post Standard. 2013. Available at: http://www.syracuse.com/news/index.ssf/2013/07/syracuses_15_homicides_more_than_last_year_if_pace_continues_2013_will_be_the_wo.html. Accessed April 18, 2016.

29. Office of Justice Research and Performance, New York State Division of Criminal Justice Services. Crime, Arrest and Firearm Activity Report: Date Reported through December 31, 2015. Issued Date: February 04, 2016.

30. Xu J, Murphy SL, Kochanek JD, et al. Deaths: Final Data for 2013. National Vital Statistics Reports; vol 64 no 2. Hyattsville, MD: National Center for Health Statistics, 2016. Available from: https://www.cdc.gov/nchs/data/nvsr/nvsr64/nvsr64_02.pdf.

31. Newgard CD, Kuppermann N, Holmes JF, et al. Gunshot injuries in children served by emergency services. Pediatrics 2013;132(5):862–70.

32. Kim D. Social determinants of health in relation to firearm-related homicides in the United States: a nationwide multilevel cross-sectional study. PLoS Med 2019;16(12). https://doi.org/10.1371/journal.pmed.1002978.

33. Knopov A, Rothman EF, Cronin SW, et al. The role of racial residential segregation in black-white disparities in firearm homicide at the state level in the United States, 1991-2015. J Natl Med Assoc 2019;111(1):62–75.

34. Goin DE, Rudolph KE, Ahern J. Predictors of firearm violence in urban communities: a machine-learning approach. Health Place 2018;51:61–7.

35. Krieger N, Feldman JM, Waterman PD, et al. Local residential segregation matters: stronger association of census tract compared to conventional city-level measures with fatal and non-fatal assaults (Total and Firearm Related), using the index of concentration at the extremes (ICE) for racial, economic, and racialized economic segregation, Massachusetts (US), 1995–2010. J Urban Health 2017;94(2):244–58.

36. Rowhani-Rahbar A, Quistberg DA, Morgan ER, et al. Income inequality and firearm homicide in the US: a county-level cohort study. Inj Prev 2019;25:i25–30.

37. Williams DR, Lawrence JA, Davis BA. Racism and health: evidence and needed research. Annu Rev Public Health 2019;40:105–25.

38. Bailey ZD, Krieger N, Agénor M, et al. America: Equity and Equality in Health 3: Structural racism and health inequities in the USA: evidence and interventions. Lancet 2017;389(10077):1453–63. Available at: www.thelancet.com/.
39. Michney TM, Winling L. New perspectives on new deal housing policy: explicating and mapping HOLC loans to African Americans. J Urban Hist 2019; 46(1):150–80.
40. Benns M, Ruther M, Nash N, et al. The impact of historical racism on modern gun violence: redlining in the city of Louisville, KY. Injury 2020. https://doi.org/10.1016/j.injury.2020.06.042.
41. Gee GC. A multilevel analysis of the relationship between institutional and individual racial discrimination and health status. Am J Public Health 2002;92:615–23.
42. Nardone A, Casey JA, Morello-Frosch R, et al. Associations between historical residential redlining and current age-adjusted rates of emergency department visits due to asthma across eight cities in California: an ecological study. Lancet Planet Health 2020;4:e24–31. Available at: www.thelancet.com/.
43. Krieger N, Van Wye G, Huynh M, et al. Structural racism, historical redlining, and risk of preterm birth in New York City, 2013-2017. Am J Public Health 2020;110(7): 1046–53.
44. Krieger N, Wright E, Chen JT, et al. Cancer stage at diagnosis, historical redlining, and current neighborhood characteristics: breast, cervical, lung, and colorectal cancer, Massachusetts, 2001-2015. Am J Epidemiol 2020. https://doi.org/10.1093/aje/kwaa045.
45. Beyer KM, Zhou Y, Matthews K, et al. New spatially continuous indices of redlining and racial bias in mortgage lending: links to survival after breast cancer diagnosis and implications for health disparities research. Health Place 2016;40(July): 34–43.
46. Lukachko A, Hatzenbuehler ML, Keyes KM. Structural racism and myocardial infarction in the United States. Soc Sci Med 2014;103:42–50.
47. Parham-Payne W. The role of the media in the disparate response to gun violence in America. J Black Stud 2014;45(8):752–68.
48. Shanahan L, Hill SN, Gaydosh LM, et al. Does despair really kill? A roadmap for an evidence-based answer. Am J Public Health 2019;109(6):854–8.
49. Case A, Deaton A. Rising morbidity and mortality in midlife among white non-Hispanic Americans in the 21st century. Proc Natl Acad Sci U S A 2015; 112(49):15078–83.
50. Case A, Deaton A. Mortality and morbidity in the 21st Century. Spring (TX): Brookings Pap Econ Act; 2017.
51. deBruyn J. Research tentatively links COVID-19 gun sales spike to increased violence. Guns and America. 2020. Available at: https://gunsandamerica.org/story/20/07/07/coronavirus-pandemic-gun-sales-violence-research/. Accessed August 4, 2020.
52. Couch KA, Fairlie RW, Xu H. The impacts of COVID-19 on minority unemployment: first evidence from April 2020 CPS Microdata. 2020. Available at: https://ssrn.com/abstract=3604814. Accessed August 4, 2020.

Rural Communities and Violence

James M. Dodington, MD[a],*, Kathleen M. O'Neill, MD[b]

KEYWORDS

- Rural youth violence prevention • Adolescent suicide • Firearm injury prevention

KEY POINTS

- Among the US geographic regions classified as rural, death rates are persistently and significantly higher for children and teens compared with their urban peers.
- Rural children and adolescents are more likely to commit suicide than their urban counterparts.
- The rate of unintentional firearm injuries is increased for rural children and teens.
- Restricting access to lethal means through safe firearm storage is one of the few proven prevention strategies found to decrease unintentional firearm injuries and suicides.

INTRODUCTION
Nature of the Problem

The impact of violence-related injuries for children and adolescents in rural communities must be examined separately from their urban counterparts, and with specific attention to race and ethnic differences in injury epidemiology. The focus of this article will be on rural populations in the United States, examining scientific studies that point to worrisome trends for rural children and teens, and discussing how rural pediatric populations suffer significantly, and need interventions built around mechanisms of injury that specifically impact their communities.

Although the overall rate of death for children in the United States has decreased over the past 2 decades, recent studies suggest that significant disparities exist within the US population, especially among racial/ethnic groups, with elevated rates of death among American Indian/Alaskan Native and non-Hispanic black children.[1] Beyond this, data indicate that, among US geographic regions classified as rural, death rates are persistently and significantly higher as compared with their urban peers and the disparity is even greater for American Indian/Alaskan Native and non-Hispanic black rural children and teens.[2,3] This disparity is not new. Its persistence and multifactorial causes however, require further research and the implementation of injury and

[a] Yale School of Medicine, 100 York Street, Suite 1F, New Haven, CT 06511, USA; [b] Investigative Medicine Program, Yale School of Medicine, 100 York Street, Suite 1F, New Haven, CT 06511, USA
* Corresponding author.
E-mail address: james.dodington@yale.edu

Pediatr Clin N Am 68 (2021) 401–412
https://doi.org/10.1016/j.pcl.2020.12.004
0031-3955/21/© 2020 Elsevier Inc. All rights reserved.

violence prevention programs. Although some factors, such as the distance to trauma centers for specialized trauma care, the closure of rural hospitals, and access to other specialty care, are concerns across the age spectrum of rural health care, specific mechanisms of injury, such as firearm suicide for adolescents, are staggering drivers of the increased death rates among rural youth and are a key point of focus for this article.[2,4,5]

DEFINITIONS
Rural Population

Although there is some variability in the classification of rural populations in the studies discussed in this article, almost all reference the US Census Bureau, which states that a rural population is composed of areas that are "not urban." In the most strict sense, this definition means less than 10,000 people but is often inclusive of "micropolitan areas," which include 10,000 to 50,000 people. These areas account for roughly 15% of the US population per the National Center for Health Statistics in a 2013 analysis.

VIOLENCE-RELATED INJURIES AND DEATH IN RURAL US CHILDREN AND ADOLESCENTS

In this article, we examine 2 instances of violence-related injury and death in rural US children and adolescents. We examine childhood violence-related injuries, with a limited discussion of child abuse and neglect, followed by an in-depth analysis of self-inflicted violent injuries, including unintentional firearm injuries and adolescent suicides, both of which have been associated with increased risks for rural children and teens.

RURAL CHILD ABUSE AND NEGLECT

In terms of violence-related injuries for rural children, an important direct form of violence against children living in rural areas in particular is inflicted injuries resulting from child abuse and injuries that result from child neglect. It is known that there are higher rates of childhood poverty in rural areas of the United States, and that increased density of poverty within a community can be associated with abusive injuries for children, shown in association with rates of abusive injuries for children covered by Medicaid insurance.[6,7] Importantly, social services are an important resource for children and families living in poverty and there is evidence that rural areas suffer from a lack of integrated social services.[8] Two studies examining the rates of hospitalization for child abuse across the rural–urban spectrum, including 1 study in Ohio and another examining the rates of hospitalized children nationally, have not shown clear elevation of risk of inflicted injuries resulting in hospitalization for children living in rural settings; in both studies, associations between poverty and increased rates of hospitalization for inflicted injury exist.[9,10] Although it is not clear that rural children face an increased rate of inflicted injury secondary to child abuse, there are mechanisms of injury that are associated with neglect, such as unintentional firearm injuries, which are frequently lethal and are associated with rural children and teens.[11–13]

UNINTENTIONAL FIREARM INJURIES IN RURAL CHILDREN AND TEENS

Firearm injuries remain a leading cause of injury and death in children, and importantly, unintentional injuries are both a significant mechanism of injury in the United States and a leading cause of injury among rural children.[11–13] Although there are limited studies on self-inflicted injuries, especially nonfatal firearm injuries in the United States, 1 study of pediatric firearm hospitalizations showed that for children ages 5 to 9 and 10 to 14 years, unintentional firearm injuries were the most common type of firearm injury and were more common in rural and micropolitan areas.[11] Linking this epidemiologic trend to violence-related injury for rural children is a finding in 2 studies that surveyed the American Academic of Pediatrics Section of Child Abuse and Neglect and a sample of members of the National Association of Social Workers, both showing that a majority of members consider access to an "unsecured and/or loaded firearm" to be a form of child neglect.[14] If one interprets these findings to mean that access to unsecured firearms is a form of child neglect, it recasts firearm safe storage as a violence prevention technique, with potential impacts on both unintentional firearm injuries and suicide prevention.

RURAL ADOLESCENT SUICIDE

Suicide is the second leading cause of death for adolescents aged 10 to 17 years old.[15] Firearms suicide is the most common method of successful suicide among adolescents. Of all successful adolescent suicides, 41% were committed with a firearm and in rural areas more than one-half of adolescent suicides were committed with a firearm (**Fig. 1**).[15] Rural children and adolescents in particular are more likely to commit suicide than their urban counterparts. In 1 study that looked at 8 years of US vital statistics data, the authors concluded that rural counties and urban counties had similar pediatric firearm mortality rates (see **Fig. 1**). However, the rural pediatric firearm mortality was largely due to suicide, with children and adolescents living in rural settings being twice as likely to die from firearm suicide as compared with their urban

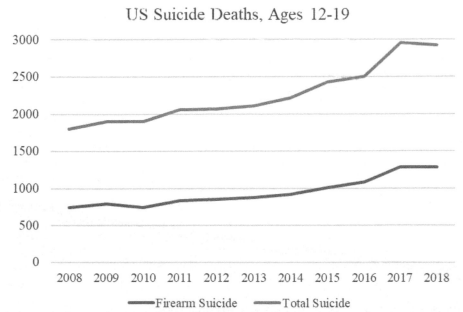

Fig. 1. US adolescent suicides and rural firearm suicide trend. (*Data from* Web-based Injury Statistics Query and Reporting System (WISQARS).2018; Available at https://www.cdc.gov/injury/wisqars/index.html. Accessed July 22nd, 2020.)

counterparts.[16] Multiple other studies have reached similar conclusions, with some suggesting that suicide rates in rural versus urban counties are increasing over time (see **Fig. 1**).[11,17,18]

RISK FACTORS FOR SUICIDE

Overall, the risk factors for adolescent suicide include both static (fixed attributes that confer a "baseline" risk) and dynamic (attributes that fluctuate through a person's life) factors. Static risk factors for adolescent suicide include age, gender, history of mental illness including previous suicide attempt, sexual orientation, and geographic location. Dynamic risk factors include meeting the criteria for a psychiatric disorder, social stress, and the presence of a gun in the home.

STATIC RISK FACTORS: ASSESSING BASELINE RISK

Children (ages 5–11 years) are at a decreased risk for suicide,[19] whereas adolescents (ages 12–19 years) are at an increased risk for death from suicide as compared with adults. The risk for adolescents increases linearly after the age of 12.[20,21] One nationally representative survey from 2015 estimated that 17.7% of US high school students seriously considered attempting suicide, 14.6% made a suicide plan, and 8.6% attempted suicide 1 or more times in the year before the survey.[22] Only approximately one-third of those attempting suicide by any means (2.8% of US high school student total) incurred an injury that required medical attention.[22]

Gender is also significantly associated with risk of suicide. Although adolescent females were more likely to have suicidal ideation, make a plan, and attempt suicide,[22] adolescent males are much more likely to successfully commit suicide.[20] Importantly, adolescent males more often choose to use a firearm as a means of suicide as compared with females.[20,23] Adolescents identifying as lesbian, gay, bisexual, or transgender are 2 to 6 times more likely to attempt suicide compared with heterosexual adolescents.[24–27] Transgender individuals have reported rates of lifetime suicide attempts of up to 52%.[28,29]

A family and personal history of psychopathology including suicide, physical or sexual abuse, and exposure to violence also constitute a major risk factor for suicide among adolescents.[23,26] Adolescents who have made a suicide attempt in the past are much more likely to commit suicide in the future, especially if they have used methods other than drug overdose or cutting (ie, firearm, drowning, falls, or hanging).[21,23,30]

Rural adolescents are at a particularly high risk for suicide despite having similar rates of depression and access to mental health resources compared with their urban counterparts.[11,16–18] One study in California found that rural adolescents were 75% less likely to have suicidal ideation and more than 80% less likely to attempt suicide compared with urban adolescents.[31] Similar results were found in other populations.[32] In that study and in others, urban and rural youth were equally likely to receive psychological services for suicidal ideation.[31–33] Nevertheless, despite a possibly decreased incidence of suicidal ideation and attempt and along with access to mental health resources similar to their urban counterparts, rural adolescents are still twice as likely to die from suicide.[17,18]

DYNAMIC RISK FACTORS: POTENTIAL FOR INTERVENTION

The majority of adolescents with suicidal ideation (>80%) meet the criteria for a psychiatric disorder.[34] The majority of those who attempt suicide have a major depressive disorder, but other psychiatric disorders include anxiety disorders, post-traumatic stress disorder, oppositional defiant disorder, eating disorder, and bipolar disorder.[34,35] Suicide attempts are often preceded by social stress including bullying, conflicts with parents, romantic breakups, and trouble in school.[19,23,36,37] Importantly, the presence of a gun in the home is independently associated with completed suicide among adolescents.[23,38]

MEANS MATTER: ACCESS TO FIREARMS INCREASES THE RISK OF SUICIDE

Firearm suicide is more lethal than other methods of suicide.[39] Firearm suicide had a case fatality rate of 82.5% in 1 publication, whereas lethal ingestion of drugs or poison had a case fatality rate of 1.5%.[39] Not only are firearms more deadly, but they also require less skill than other means to be used successfully.

Ecological and Case Control Studies: Where There Are More Guns, There Are More Suicides

Over the last 3 decades, multiple studies have demonstrated that where there are more firearms, there are more suicides. One 2007 ecological study compared the rate of suicide with the percentage of individuals living in households with firearms (firearm prevalence) using state-level data. They found that a 1-percentage point absolute difference in household firearm prevalence was associated with a 1.4% increase in the rate of suicide overall and a 3.5% increase in the rate of firearm suicide specifically.[40] There was no significant difference in the rate of nonfirearm suicide. This relationship was upheld even after adjustment for serious mental illness, poverty, alcohol and substance use disorder, and unemployment. When stratified by age and sex, there were almost twice as many completed suicides in the states with a high gun prevalence for all age groups and sexes as compared with states with the lowest gun prevalence, with the highest rate ratio for firearm suicides in the youngest age group (5–19 years).[40] Other ecological studies looking at firearm prevalence and suicide rates have come to similar conclusions.[41,42]

A case control study of adolescents who committed suicide in Colorado found that adolescents who committed suicide had almost a 4 times increased odds of access to firearms in their homes compared with their age- and sex-matched controls (odds ratio, 3.9; 95% confidence interval, 1.11–13.8), even after adjustment for significant risk factors.[43] Case control studies looking at suicides in all age groups have also come to similar conclusions.[44,45]

PREVENTING ACCESS TO LETHAL MEANS WILL SAVE LIVES

The availability of lethal means is associated with the suicide rate of a given region. In the United States, firearms are the most common means of suicide.[46,47] Given that there is an association between access to lethal means and suicide, restricting access to lethal means or decreasing the lethality of suicidal behavior is an effective suicide prevention strategy.[48–52]

One of the strongest risk factors for dying from suicide is a previous suicide attempt.[21,23,30] However, many adolescents who successfully commit suicide will not have this risk factor. Overall, 60% of those who die from suicide have never had a previous attempt.[53] Among adolescents, this number increases to about 75%.[38,54,55] Given that firearm suicide has the highest case fatality rate of all methods of suicide, decreasing access to this lethal means could save lives by allowing for secondary prevention after an unsuccessful suicide attempt.[39]

Although improving access to mental health care across the United States is an important strategy for suicide prevention in general, the increased rate of suicide in rural areas is likely impacted by many other factors, including increased access to lethal means, such as firearms. Restricting access to lethal means is one of the few proven prevention strategies found to decrease suicides at the population level.[56,57]

KEY STRATEGIES TO DECREASING ADOLESCENT SUICIDE

Overall, experts recommend the following strategies for adolescent suicide prevention.

- *Education:* Although few public education campaigns have been systematically evaluated through targeted research, decreasing the stigma and increasing the awareness of risk factors for suicide and mental illness remain important suicide prevention strategies. Specifically, educational campaigns for physicians and adults who regularly work with children show promise for reducing suicidal behavior. At a population level, mental illness is undertreated in the primary care setting.[58–60] Approximately two-thirds of younger individuals who commit suicide have had contact with a physician within 1 year of death, and 1 in 5 saw a physician in the month preceding their death.[61] There is some evidence to support the effectiveness of improving access to evidence-based depression treatment for adolescents in preventing suicidal behavior.[62] This factor represents an opportunity for prevention efforts in the primary care setting.
- *Screening:* Although there is insufficient evidence to support the routine use of screening for suicide in all adolescents,[63] the American Academy of Pediatrics recommends that pediatricians ask questions about depression, suicidal thoughts, mood disorders, bullying, sexual orientation, and other risk factors in their routine history taking at health maintenance visits.[64] For those adolescents perceived to be at risk, there are a number of validated screening tools for depression and suicide validated in adolescents.[65,66] The American Academy of Pediatrics also recommends routinely discussing the risk of adolescent suicide with parents and specifically asking about whether firearms are kept in the home.[64]
- *Intense follow-up care after suicide attempts:* Approximately one-quarter of adolescents who attempt suicide will make another attempt in the next 5 years and up to 8% will ultimately die by suicide.[67] Therefore, intensive follow-up care after a suicide attempt is an important secondary prevention strategy for adolescent suicide.
- *Decrease access to lethal means:* As reviewed elsewhere in this article.

COMPREHENSIVE FIREARM HARM REDUCTION: SAFE STORAGE

The most effective way for parents to protect their children against firearm injuries, both unintentional and intentional, is to not have a firearm in the home. For families who maintain a firearm in the home, which is more common in rural households, the risk of a firearm injury can be mitigated through the implementation of safe storage practices. Multiple studies demonstrate that unsafe firearm storage practices significantly increase the risk associated with firearm injury and successful suicide.[68]

In particular for children and adolescents, the risk of firearm injury is lower when firearms are stored unloaded and locked with either a safe or a gunlock (**Fig. 2**).[69,70] Despite this finding, parents often do not store their firearms properly. Of all gun owners living with children, 20% store at least 1 firearm unlocked and loaded.[71]

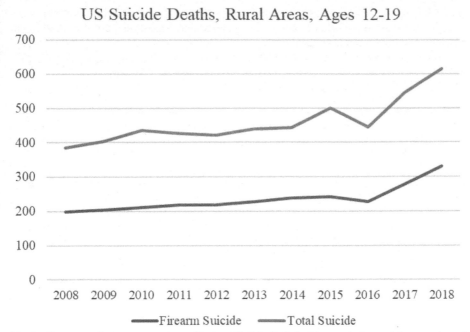

US Suicide Deaths, Rural Areas, Ages 12-19

Firearm Suicide   Total Suicide

Fig. 2. Firearm safe storage options. (Project ChildSafe Safe Storage infographic reproduced with permission from National Shooting Sports Foundation.)

Among all gun owners in one 1 , 45% stored at least 1 gun unlocked and 54% stored at least 1 gun loaded.[72] Firearm storage practices do not differ between households with and without a history of mental illness.[73] Promoting or requiring safe storage practices for all firearms in a household with children and teens is an important firearm injury prevention strategy across the United States, but particularly in rural areas.

Safety Devices Are Critical to Safe Firearm Storage: Counseling Patients and Families

The practice of safe firearm storage requires patients and families to choose from various devices to secure their firearm and to prevent unintended use (see **Fig. 2**). In terms of firearm safety devices, there are limited scientific studies on the effectiveness and use of specific devices.

In terms of community preferences for a safety device as it relates to rural populations, a study in rural Alaska examined whether the installation of gun cabinets (installed gun safes) improved firearm storage practices. The study authors concluded that installed gun safes may be important to safe storage practices in communities with high levels of gun ownership and unlocked firearms in rural communities.[74]

SUMMARY AND RECOMMENDATIONS

Given the epidemiologic trend of persistently elevated death rates for rural children and teens, and the known increased rate of firearm injuries and adolescent suicides specifically in rural areas, the United States needs a national strategy for rural pediatric injury and violence prevention.[2] More research needs to be done to better understand the most effective strategies for prevention. Currently, research has demonstrated that some of the most promising interventions include improved screening and coordination of social services for child abuse and neglect prevention, lethal means restriction to decrease adolescent suicide, increasing awareness among adults who regularly work with children (teachers, clergy, etc), and education for medical professionals to be aware of risks and increase screening when appropriate.[48]

CLINICS CARE POINTS

- The rates of unintentional firearm injuries are higher for rural children and teens and clinicians should educate themselves on firearm safety devices and potentially procure devices to be distributed in the clinical setting to support safety messaging to patients and families.

- Rural children and adolescents are more likely to die by suicide than their urban counterparts and counseling interventions in the clinical setting should take this risk factor into consideration.

- Restricting access to lethal means through safe firearm storage is one of the few proven prevention strategies found to decrease suicides, and clinicians should education themselves on suicide prevention resources in their community and use firearm safety promotion as a means to support suicide prevention in rural communities.

DISCLOSURE

The authors have nothing to disclose.

REFERENCES

1. Khan SQ, Berrington de Gonzalez A, Best AF, et al. Infant and youth mortality trends by race/ethnicity and cause of death in the United States. JAMA Pediatr 2018;172(12):e183317.
2. Probst J, Zahnd W, Breneman C. Declines in pediatric mortality fall short for rural US children. Health Aff (Millwood) 2019;38(12):2069–76.
3. Singh GK, Siahpush M. Widening rural-urban disparities in life expectancy, U.S., 1969-2009. Am J Prev Med 2014;46(2):e19–29.
4. Hale N, Probst J, Robertson A. Rural area deprivation and hospitalizations among children for ambulatory care sensitive conditions. J Community Health 2016; 41(3):451–60.
5. Hsia RY, Shen YC. Rising closures of hospital trauma centers disproportionately burden vulnerable populations. Health Aff (Millwood) 2011;30(10):1912–20.
6. Leventhal JM, Martin KD, Gaither JR. Using US data to estimate the incidence of serious physical abuse in children. Pediatrics 2012;129(3):458–64.
7. Wang M, Kleit RG, Cover J, et al. Spatial variations in US poverty: beyond metropolitan and non-metropolitan. Urban Stud 2012;49(3):563–85.
8. Belanger K, Stone W. The social service divide: service availability and accessibility in rural versus urban counties and impact on child welfare outcomes. Child Welfare 2008;87(4):101–24.
9. Anderson BL, Pomerantz WJ, Gittelman MA. Intentional injuries in young Ohio children: is there urban/rural variation? J Trauma Acute Care Surg 2014;77(3 Suppl 1):S36–40.
10. Puls HT, Bettenhausen JL, Markham JL, et al. Urban-rural residence and child physical abuse hospitalizations: a national incidence study. J Pediatr 2019;205: 230–235 e232.

11. Herrin BR, Gaither JR, Leventhal JM, et al. Rural versus urban hospitalizations for firearm injuries in children and adolescents. Pediatrics 2018;142(2).
12. Monuteaux MC, Mannix R, Fleegler EW, et al. Predictors and outcomes of pediatric firearm injuries treated in the emergency department: differences by mechanism of intent. Acad Emerg Med 2016;23(7):790–5.
13. Solnick SJ, Hemenway D. Unintentional firearm deaths in the United States 2005-2015. Inj Epidemiol 2019;6:42.
14. Jennissen CA, Evans EM, Karsjens AA, et al. Social workers' determination of when children's access or potential access to loaded firearms constitutes child neglect. Inj Epidemiol 2019;6(Suppl 1):29.
15. Web-based Injury Statistics Query and Reporting System (WISQARS). 2017. Available at: https://www.cdc.gov/injury/wisqars/index.html. Accessed July 16, 2019.
16. Nance ML, Carr BG, Kallan MJ, et al. Variation in pediatric and adolescent firearm mortality rates in rural and urban US counties. Pediatrics 2010;125(6):1112–8.
17. Fontanella CA, Hiance-Steelesmith DL, Phillips GS, et al. Widening rural-urban disparities in youth suicides, United States, 1996-2010. JAMA Pediatr 2015; 169(5):466–73.
18. Singh GK, Azuine RE, Siahpush M, et al. All-cause and cause-specific mortality among US youth: socioeconomic and rural-urban disparities and international patterns. J Urban Health 2013;90(3):388–405.
19. Bridge JA, Asti L, Horowitz LM, et al. Suicide trends among elementary school-aged children in the United States From 1993 to 2012. JAMA Pediatr 2015; 169(7):673–7.
20. Sullivan EM, Annest JL, Simon TR, et al. Suicide trends among persons aged 10-24 years -United States, 1994-2012. MMWR Morb Mortal Wkly Rep 2015;64(8): 201–5.
21. Goldston DB, Daniel SS, Erkanli A, et al. Suicide attempts in a longitudinal sample of adolescents followed through adulthood: evidence of escalation. J Consult Clin Psychol 2015;83(2):253–64.
22. Kann L, McManus T, Harris WA, et al. Youth risk behavior surveillance - United States, 2015. MMWR Surveill Summ 2016;65(6):1–174.
23. Brent DA, Baugher M, Bridge J, et al. Age- and sex-related risk factors for adolescent suicide. J Am Acad Child Adolesc Psychiatry 1999;38(12):1497–505.
24. Taliaferro LA, Muehlenkamp JJ. Risk and protective factors that distinguish adolescents who attempt suicide from those who only consider suicide in the past year. Suicide Life Threat Behav 2014;44(1):6–22.
25. Jiang Y, Perry DK, Hesser JE. Adolescent suicide and health risk behaviors: Rhode Island's 2007 youth risk behavior survey. Am J Prev Med 2010;38(5): 551–5.
26. Spirito A, Esposito-Smythers C. Attempted and completed suicide in adolescence. Annu Rev Clin Psychol 2006;2:237–66.
27. Gould MS, Greenberg T, Velting DM, et al. Youth suicide risk and preventive interventions: a review of the past 10 years. J Am Acad Child Adolesc Psychiatry 2003;42(4):386–405.
28. Haas AP, Lane A. Collecting sexual orientation and gender identity data in suicide and other violent deaths: a step towards identifying and addressing LGBT mortality disparities. LGBT health 2015;2(1):84–7.
29. Mustanski B, Liu RT. A longitudinal study of predictors of suicide attempts among lesbian, gay, bisexual, and transgender youth. Arch Sex Behav 2013;42(3): 437–48.

30. Miller M, Hempstead K, Nguyen T, et al. Method choice in nonfatal self-harm as a predictor of subsequent episodes of self-harm and suicide: implications for clinical practice. Am J Public Health 2013;103(6):e61–8.
31. Goldman-Mellor S, Allen K, Kaplan MS. Rural/Urban disparities in adolescent nonfatal suicidal ideation and suicide attempt: a population-based study. Suicide Life Threat Behav 2018;48(6):709–19.
32. Margerison CE, Goldman-Mellor S. Association between rural residence and nonfatal suicidal behavior among California adults: a population-based study. J Rural Health 2019;35(2):262–9.
33. Rost K, Zhang M, Fortney J, et al. Rural-urban differences in depression treatment and suicidality. Med Care 1998;36(7):1098–107.
34. Nock MK, Green JG, Hwang I, et al. Prevalence, correlates, and treatment of lifetime suicidal behavior among adolescents: results from the National comorbidity survey replication adolescent supplement. JAMA psychiatry 2013;70(3):300–10.
35. Hoertel N, Franco S, Wall MM, et al. Mental disorders and risk of suicide attempt: a national prospective study. Mol Psychiatry 2015;20(6):718–26.
36. Sheftall AH, Asti L, Horowitz LM, et al. Suicide in elementary school-aged children and early adolescents. Pediatrics 2016;138(4).
37. Mayes SD, Baweja R, Calhoun SL, et al. Suicide ideation and attempts and bullying in children and adolescents: psychiatric and general population samples. Crisis 2014;35(5):301–9.
38. Brent DA, Perper JA, Moritz G, et al. Firearms and adolescent suicide. A community case-control study. Am J Dis Child 1993;147(10):1066–71.
39. Spicer RS, Miller TR. Suicide acts in 8 states: incidence and case fatality rates by demographics and method. Am J Public Health 2000;90(12):1885–91.
40. Miller M, Lippmann SJ, Azrael D, et al. Household firearm ownership and rates of suicide across the 50 United States. J Trauma 2007;62(4):1029–34, discussion 1034–025.
41. Hemenway D, Miller M. Association of rates of household handgun ownership, lifetime major depression, and serious suicidal thoughts with rates of suicide across US census regions. Inj Prev 2002;8(4):313–6.
42. Siegel M, Rothman EF. Firearm ownership and suicide rates among US men and women, 1981-2013. Am J Public Health 2016;106(7):1316–22.
43. Shah S, Hoffman RE, Wake L, et al. Adolescent suicide and household access to firearms in Colorado: results of a case-control study. J Adolesc Health 2000; 26(3):157–63.
44. Kellermann AL, Rivara FP, Somes G, et al. Suicide in the home in relation to gun ownership. N Engl J Med 1992;327(7):467–72.
45. Wiebe DJ. Homicide and suicide risks associated with firearms in the home: a national case-control study. Ann Emerg Med 2003;41(6):771–82.
46. Centers for Disease Control and Prevention, Web-based Injury Statistics Query and Reporting System (WISQARS), "Fatal Injury Reports". Available at: https://www.cdc.gov/injury/wisqars. Accessed July 1, 2020.
47. Ajdacic-Gross V, Weiss MG, Ring M, et al. Methods of suicide: international suicide patterns derived from the WHO mortality database. Bull World Health Organ 2008;86(9):726–32.
48. Mann JJ, Apter A, Bertolote J, et al. Suicide prevention strategies: a systematic review. JAMA 2005;294(16):2064–74.
49. Miller M, Azrael D, Barber C. Suicide mortality in the United States: the importance of attending to method in understanding population-level disparities in the burden of suicide. Annu Rev Public Health 2012;33;393 100.

50. Johnson RM, Coyne-Beasley T. Lethal means reduction: what have we learned? Curr Opin Pediatr 2009;21(5):635–40.
51. Houtsma C, Butterworth SE, Anestis MD. Firearm suicide: pathways to risk and methods of prevention. Curr Opin Psychol 2018;22:7–11.
52. Florentine JB, Crane C. Suicide prevention by limiting access to methods: a review of theory and practice. Soc Sci Med 2010;70(10):1626–32.
53. Cavanagh JT, Carson AJ, Sharpe M, et al. Psychological autopsy studies of suicide: a systematic review. Psychol Med 2003;33(3):395–405.
54. Brent DA, Perper JA, Moritz G, et al. Psychiatric risk factors for adolescent suicide: a case-control study. J Am Acad Child Adolesc Psychiatry 1993;32(3): 521–9.
55. Shaffer D, Gould MS, Fisher P, et al. Psychiatric diagnosis in child and adolescent suicide. Arch Gen Psychiatry 1996;53(4):339–48.
56. Carrington PJ. Gender, gun control, suicide and homicide in Canada. Arch Suicide Res 1999;5(1):71–5.
57. Bridges FS. Gun control law (Bill C-17), suicide, and homicide in Canada. Psychol Rep 2004;94(3 I):819–26.
58. Hirschfeld RM, Keller MB, Panico S, et al. The national depressive and manic-depressive association consensus statement on the undertreatment of depression. JAMA 1997;277(4):333 -40.
59. Jencks SF. Recognition of mental distress and diagnosis of mental disorder in primary care. JAMA 1985;253(13):1903–7.
60. Forman-Hoffman VL, Viswanathan M. Screening for depression in pediatric primary care. Curr Psychiatry Rep 2018;20(8):62.
61. Luoma JB, Martin CE, Pearson JL. Contact with mental health and primary care providers before suicide: a review of the evidence. Am J Psychiatry 2002;159(6): 909–16.
62. Asarnow JR, Jaycox LH, Duan N, et al. Effectiveness of a quality improvement intervention for adolescent depression in primary care clinics: a randomized controlled trial. JAMA 2005;293(3):311–9.
63. LeFevre ML. Screening for suicide risk in adolescents, adults, and older adults in primary care: U.S. Preventive Services Task Force recommendation statement. Ann Intern Med 2014;160(10):719–26.
64. Shain B. Suicide and suicide attempts in adolescents. Pediatrics 2016;138(1).
65. Shaffer D, Scott M, Wilcox H, et al. The Columbia Suicide Screen: validity and reliability of a screen for youth suicide and depression. J Am Acad Child Adolesc Psychiatry 2004;43(1):71–9.
66. Allgaier AK, Pietsch K, Frühe B, et al. Screening for depression in adolescents: validity of the patient health questionnaire in pediatric care. Depress anxiety 2012;29(10):906–13.
67. Owens D, Horrocks J, House A. Fatal and non-fatal repetition of self-harm. Systematic review. Br J Psychiatry 2002;181:193–9.
68. Shenassa ED, Rogers ML, Spalding KL, et al. Safer storage of firearms at home and risk of suicide: a study of protective factors in a nationally representative sample. J Epidemiol Community Health 2004;58(10):841–8.
69. Grossman DC, Mueller BA, Riedy C, et al. Gun storage practices and risk of youth suicide and unintentional firearm injuries. JAMA 2005;293(6):707–14.
70. Grossman DC, Reay DT, Baker SA. Self-inflicted and unintentional firearm injuries among children and adolescents: the source of the firearm. Arch Pediatr Adolesc Med 1999;153(8):875–8.

71. Azrael D, Cohen J, Salhi C, et al. Firearm storage in gun-owning households with children: results of a 2015 national survey. J Urban Health 2018;95(3):295–304.

72. Crifasi CK, Doucette ML, McGinty EE, et al. Storage practices of US Gun owners in 2016. Am J Public Health 2018;108(4):532–7.

73. Simonetti JA, Theis MK, Rowhani-Rahbar A, et al. Firearm storage practices in households of adolescents with and without mental illness. J Adolesc Health 2017;61(5):583–90.

74. Grossman DC, Stafford HA, Koepsell TD, et al. Improving firearm storage in Alaska native villages: a randomized trial of household gun cabinets. Am J Public Health 2012;102(Suppl 2):S291–7.

K–12 School Shootings

Implications for Policy, Prevention, and Child Well-Being

Paul M. Reeping, MS[a],*, Ariana N. Gobaud, MPH[a],
Charles C. Branas, PhD[a], Sonali Rajan, EdD[a,b]

KEYWORDS

- School shootings • School safety • School violence • Gun violence
- Active shootings • Mass shootings

KEY POINTS

- All children in K–12 schools have a right to a safe and secure learning environment, which allows for their healthy development.
- When a school shooting occurs, the harm goes beyond those who were directly injured or killed and has mental health consequences for all who are directly or indirectly affiliated with the tragedy.
- Many existing interventions—including physical security measures, active shooter drills, arming teachers, behavioral interventions, and federal or local laws—have been proposed and/or subsequently implemented without consideration for how such interventions may have an impact on the well-being of children.

INTRODUCTION

On December 14, 2012, a 20-year-old man, not yet legally old enough to carry a handgun, would go on to commit the deadliest K–12 school shooting in US history.[1] Earlier in the morning, he first murdered his mother, a firearms enthusiast, and stole her Bushmaster XM15-E2S rifle, Izhmash Canta-12 12-gauge shotgun, SIG Sauer P226, and Glock 20SF handgun, all of which were bought legally.[2] He then drove 10 minutes away to Sandy Hook Elementary School in Newtown, Connecticut, a kindergarten through fourth grade elementary school, where more than 400 were students enrolled. The school had security measures in place; for example, visitors needed to be

[a] Department of Epidemiology, Columbia University, Mailman School of Public Health, 722 West 168th Street, New York, NY 10032, USA; [b] Department of Health and Behavior Studies, Columbia University, Teachers College, 525 West 120th Street, 530F Thorndike Hall, Box 114, New York, NY 10027, USA
* Corresponding author. Department of Epidemiology, Mailman School of Public Health, Columbia University, 722 West 168th Street, New York, NY 10032.
E-mail address: pmr2149@cumc.columbia.edu

Pediatr Clin N Am 68 (2021) 413–426
https://doi.org/10.1016/j.pcl.2020.12.005
0031-3955/21/© 2020 Elsevier Inc. All rights reserved.

identified and buzzed into the building, which was locked once the school day began.[1] Using the Bushmaster rifle, the perpetrator bypassed this system by shooting through plate glass in the front of the school. After killing the principal and school psychologist and wounding a teacher who tried to stop the attack, he opened fire on 2 first-grade classrooms.[1] In 1 of the classrooms, he shot and killed a teacher and behavioral specialist who had attempted to shelter the students in the bathroom. He then murdered all the students except a 6-year-old girl; she survived by hiding in the corner of the bathroom and playing dead, likely underneath her murdered classmates. Fifteen children perished in this classroom.[1] In the second classroom, the teacher and special needs teacher put themselves between the perpetrator and the children, and several students were able to escape the room when the shooter reloaded his firearm. Tragically, 5 students still were killed, including both teachers. Within approximately 6 minutes, 20 children (only 6–7 years old) and 6 adults were killed before the gunman committed suicide using the handgun.[1] This tragedy relaunched a national conversation about the occurrence of mass shootings, specifically the physical, psychological, and educational harm inflicted on children. Despite being touted as the "tipping point" in gun violence prevention,[3] only individual states have been successful in passing legislation in hopes of reducing mass shootings. To this day, there has not been significant legislation passed at the federal level to prevent these incidents from occurring in the future.[4]

Using the most commonly used definition of a mass shooting—an incident where 4 or more individuals are killed by a single (or sometimes pair) of perpetrators[5]—studies have found that children and teens (individuals under the age of 18) make up a surprisingly high percentage of the victims killed in these tragedies. In 2019, children comprised 22% of the population in the United States[6] and accounted for approximately 25% of victims in all mass shootings.[7] Children are even more likely to be victimized with a gun if the event occurs in the home. Between 2009 and 2016, there were 102 mass shootings, of which 71 occurred in the home and 31 in public. Children under the age of 18 accounted for nearly half (44%) of the deaths in domestic mass shootings and 10% of the victims in public mass shootings.[8]

Although children and teens usually are not targeted in public mass shootings,[8] school shootings in K–12 schools—which include mass shootings—remain an unfortunate exception. These tragedies have an impact primarily on children and teens and are especially concerning given the age of the victims. The definition of a school shooting, like mass shootings, can vary widely, ranging from an accidental discharge of a gun at school, to the injury or death of a student by a firearm, and to a school mass shooting.[9] Using the definition of any incident of interpersonal gunfire in a K–12 school, the *Washington Post* created a data set that details any school shooting since the Columbine School shooting, in 1999.[10] Using these data, the number of school shootings per year, with some of the most infamous school shootings labeled, is presented in **Fig. 1**. Regardless of how a school shooting is defined, all of these events can have detrimental effects on a child's well-being, development, and critical learning outcomes. This is evident particularly if considering that school shootings have an impact not only on those children who are physically injured and killed but also on those who witness the shooting, hear gunshots, or know a friend or family member who was killed, among other levels of exposure.[11] Indeed, the short-term and long-term implications of school shootings on communities across the United States can be devastating.[12,13]

K–12 school shootings are of particular interest given the expectation of safety within a school's walls and the right of every child to learn and thrive in a safe school environment. An apt comparison can be made between school shootings and plane crashes. Deaths due to both are rare,[14,15] and planes and classrooms also are presumed to be safe places. Due to the presumption of safety, however, if something

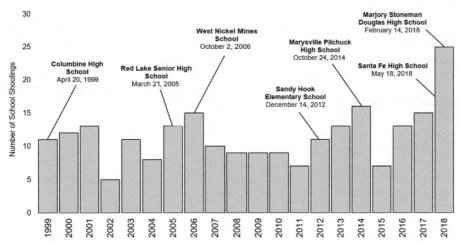

Fig. 1. Number of school shootings in the United States since the Columbine High School shooting.

goes wrong, the event rightfully is seen not only as tragic but also as preventable. As a result, both are more likely to make international news than more frequent tragedies, such as car crashes or domestic shootings.[16,17] This heightened media response may be a reason why many are terrified of these events; in 2018, Americans rated mass shootings, including school shootings, as the second most important event of the year (with the first being the economy).[18] And the impact of a school shooting may feel particularly devastating, because schools are intended to be safe spaces within which children should be able to thrive and foster their physical, social, and emotional development. The notion that schools could be the site of such violence is counter to understanding—and expectations of—what schools can and should be. At the same time, an argument can be made that the fear associated with the anticipation of gun violence in schools also is due to a loss of control by the victims.[19] Just as a passenger on a plane has no way of preventing a mechanical dysfunction or error by the pilot, a parent has little ability to stop a school shooting in the moment. Importantly, however, the 2 scenarios differ in the way society responds to them. Despite how rare plane crashes prove to be, if one occurs, there is an immediate investigation and steps are made to prevent a future occurrence with significant investments of money and research. The airline industry continues to produce safer airplanes, stricter safety regulations, and a commitment to bringing the number of the accidents to zero. This same mentality should exist with shootings in schools—they are tragedies that should not exist in modern society. Yet, the number of school mass shootings, which had been relatively consistent year-to-year since the 1999 Columbine High School mass shooting, has started to increase in incidence since 2015.[9] Data indicate that more mass school shootings occurred in K–12 schools in 2017 than any other year.[9] Furthermore, the solutions to preventing a school shooting are not as straightforward as preventing a mechanical failure in a machine, because they need to consider the mental and educational well-being of children.

HARM BEYOND INJURY AND DEATH

Research has confirmed that the implications of youth being exposed to gun violence—in particular, a school shooting—can occur even if no one is killed or injured.[11] For example, a significant body of work has demonstrated that the anticipation of violence more generally can lead to heightened anxiety, fear, and depression across a range of populations.[20-22] According to the *Washington Post*, well over 200 instances of gunfire in K–12 schools have occurred in the United States in the 20 years since the Columbine shooting in Colorado,[10] the most publicly notable being mass shooting tragedies at schools like Sandy Hook Elementary School and Marjory Stoneman Douglas High School. Although approximately 150 students and educators have been killed and 300 injured by mass shootings in schools, more than 236,000 students have been exposed to gun violence at their K–12 school since Columbine.[10] The number of students exposed to interpersonal gunfire in their schools per year is presented in **Fig. 2**.[10] This number, however, is still an underestimate of the total harm created by these events because the reactions and responses to the school mass shootings also could have negative mental health outcomes for children across the United States through anxiety of the anticipation that a shooting might take place at their school in the future.

For example, the hundreds of thousands of students who may have avoided being physically injured by a firearm during these attacks still may experience long-term mental health consequences. Any sense of security or safety in their schools—an essential component of learning[23]—can be disrupted with insecurity after these tragedies. A review by Lowe and Galea,[24] published in 2017, examined 49 articles covering 15 mass shootings, 4 of which were in K–12 settings. Among these articles, the most common psychological outcomes that were assessed and found elevated among this population were posttraumatic stress disorder and major depression, although evidence of generalized anxiety disorder, acute stress disorder, alcohol-related conditions, drug use disorder, panic disorder, adjustment disorder, and antisocial personality disorder also were found to be significant in individuals' lives who had been affected by a mass shooting.[24] Although psychological conditions were found

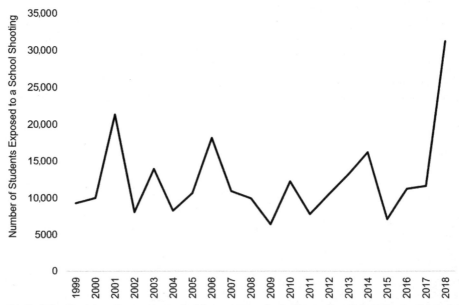

Fig. 2. Number of students exposed to interpersonal gunfire in the United States since the Columbine High School shooting.

more severe for those who had greater exposure (ie, witnessing the attack or knowing a victim), those with little direct exposure to the shooting still had at least short-term mental distress of some kind following the incident.[24] Furthermore, although this review included both adults and minors, children and teens who were exposed to these events often experienced higher rates of psychological disorders, including posttraumatic stress disorder, in comparison to their adult counterparts. In another study, depending on the way in which they are exposed, approximately 30% to 40% of children who are exposed to a life-threatening event develop symptoms of posttraumatic stress disorder.[25] In some cases, mental anguish, often fueled by survivor's guilt and trauma,[26] can result in deaths years after the incident. For example, 2 Marjory Stoneman Douglas High School students committed suicide a little over a year after the school mass shooting, and a father of a Sandy Hook Elementary School victim committed suicide in 2019.[27,28]

Gun violence in K–12 schools persists, with potentially devastating and traumatic implications for communities around the United States. The following sections present evidence in support of several solutions at multiple levels for this endemic, while also evaluating the lack of evidence that exists for other solutions that currently are in place.

SOLUTIONS AND GAPS IN EVIDENCE

Like all public health crises, the solution to the persistence of gun violence in K–12 schools will require a multifaceted and coordinated effort that draws on a wide range of evidence-informed strategies and involves multiple stakeholders. Importantly, these solutions also must consider the well-being of children in their approach. This section identifies examples of current approaches to gun violence prevention in schools and speaks to their strengths and limitations.

School Level

Physical security measures

The image of a school has changed since the 1999 Columbine shooting in Littleton, Colorado, with the implementation of security measures, such as metal detectors, armed guards, and zero-tolerance policies.[29] In 1999, less than 20% of schools had security cameras; now, more than 80% do.[29] These policies also disproportionately affect schools in communities with a lower socioeconomic status and where the primary population are students of color—regardless of crime rates—and are 1 facet of the school-to-prison pipeline.[30,31] Unfortunately, evidence surrounding these policies is limited and, when available, conflicting. Some researchers have found that more security measures in school, such as metal detectors and armed guards, resulted in students feeling less safe compared with schools without these measures.[32–34] Other researchers have reported the opposite: students felt more safe with these policies[35] or that these security measures have little effect on academic performance.[36] Furthermore, although there is evidence in support of some behavior interventions in preventing school violence, such as counseling, mentoring, and peer mediation,[37–39] most studies evaluating physical security policies have been inconclusive.[40] This dilemma proposes a problem: school districts not only are implementing policies that have not been proved effective in reducing violence but also are doing so without knowing the mental health consequences of these measures. The lives significantly influenced by school shootings are vast and uncountable; therefore, research on the best ways to reduce harm related to these tragedies, both mental and physical, is critical.

Lockdowns and active shooter drills

In the weeks before the school shooting at Sandy Hook Elementary School, the school had practiced lockdown and safety procedures; it is thought that the shooter bypassed one of the first-grade classrooms because the teacher had forgotten to remove black construction paper from the window of the classroom door.[1] In the years following, lockdown and active shooting drills have increased in American schools: according to the National Center for Education Statistics, approximately 95% of schools now conduct these drills.[41] These drills are meant to help students and teachers practice quickly locking the door and windows/blinds, finding cover in a classroom, and remaining quiet and, in some instances, include multioptional responses, such as teaching students and educators how to create barricades, evacuate the school, and actively resist a shooter.[42] Simulation studies have shown that lockdowns, in particular, multioptional ones, may save lives.[42] But the implementation of these drills is not without controversy, because there is fear that they might by harmful for a child's emotional and mental well-being,[43] can be used to the shooter's advantage,[44] or may numb students' reactions if a real shooting were to occur.[45] One survey among students between the ages of 14 and 24 found that although 56% reported that they do help to teach students what to do in case of an attack, 60% of the 815 respondents reported that the drill made them feel "scared and hopeless."[46] It, therefore, is important that these drills are implemented appropriately. For example, if the drills are well planned and the students are warned about the drill before it happens (as opposed to being surprised), some of the harm from these practices could be avoided.[47] Even so, school psychologists should be included in both the planning and aftermath of active shooter drills to prevent trauma from occurring, especially with students of younger ages.[48]

Arming teachers

The shooting at Marjory Stoneman Douglas High School in Parkland, Florida, reignited a national conversation around arming teachers with firearms. Although not a new idea, it brought this concept to the forefront of the national discourse. Unfortunately, and as recent work has illustrated, little is known about the effectiveness of arming teachers in deterring gun violence in schools,[49] including how its implementation would work. For example, many law enforcement officers receive more than 800 hours of basic training, which includes 168 hours of training specifically on weapon use, self-defense tactics, and the use of force.[50] States that have laws, however, aimed at arming school personnel offer significantly less training—if any—to their school staff.[49] Research also suggests that arming teachers could heighten levels of anxiety and negatively affect a school's climate as opposed to serving as an effective deterrence of gun violence.[51] A large majority of teachers and parents are opposed to the idea as well. A recent survey of 500 US teachers found that 73% opposed proposals to arm school staff,[52] and a survey of parents of elementary, middle, and high school students found that 63% oppose arming teachers.[53] Arming teachers also would require a contingency plan in place for all possible firearm-related scenarios (whether intentional or accidental), an understanding about the implications of this proposed effort on teacher burden and burnout, a clear sense of how this would resonate or possibly conflict with existing school policies, and an exorbitant cost investment.[49,54]

Efforts to address early antecedents of violent behavior

The prevention of engagement in violence behavior among children—in particular, adolescents—has a long and complicated history. As a health crisis, gun violence in schools and its related behavioral antecedents should be addressed, not solely or primarily with punitive measures. In today's school environment, children often are viewed either as perpetrators to be punished or as victims to be protected without building on their agency.[55] Investing in evidence-based preventive efforts that are intended to promote critical skill development, however, and doing so in ways that recognize the resources and agency that children and adolescents bring to the issue, likely are far more effective ways both to address the perceived threat of gun violence and prevent the onset of violent tendencies among youth, while also promoting well-being more broadly. For example, skill-oriented initiatives with a social-emotional learning focus have been shown to help youth develop healthier coping mechanisms and improve capabilities to address and manage social anxieties, interpersonal conflict with peers and sexual partners, feelings of anger or frustration, challenges with emotion regulation, and engagement in aggressive behaviors.[56] Investing in such efforts early on in the developmental trajectory has the potential to be effective, because research demonstrates that experiences with violence beget more violence.[57] In line with work in developmental epidemiology,[58,59] the authors anticipate that prevention strategies that reduce the onset of more minor incidents of violence among youth (hypothesized to be early antecedents of gun violence), in turn may prevent incidents of gun violence. Other school-based and classroom-based initiatives focused on the school climate[60–62] and engaging parents in the school community[63] also have been shown to have an impact on reducing aggressive and violent behaviors more broadly. At the same time, work on positive youth development programs have identified short-term impacts on reducing violent outcomes, but the long-term efficacy of such efforts is not clear.[64] Much of this work also has elucidated that more research is needed to better understand the efficacy of such preventive efforts on reducing gun violence in schools.[63] But these efforts can and should be considered part of a broader menu of strategies that schools pursue as they consider how best to keep their communities safe.

Bullying and warning signs

A majority of K–12 school mass shootings are perpetrated by minors,[9] and, in many incidences, research has found that bullying—both being the target of or committing the bullying—is a major risk factor for committing school based violence.[65] An evaluation of 15 mass shootings found that 13 of the perpetrators had experienced acute or chronic rejection.[66] For example, in a case of the Sandy Hook mass shooting, the gunman had been described as "very withdrawn emotionally" and "quiet and socially awkward."[67] In response to these commonalities between the perpetrators, Sandy Hook Promise, an organization with a mission to "create a culture engaged in preventing shootings, violence, and other harmful acts in schools," developed the Start With Hello program and curriculum.[68] The goal of this program is to teach students to be more socially inclusive of one another, with hope that this will reduce bullying and rejection that some students might experience.

In many cases of school violence, there often also are warning signs preceding the event. A study conducted by the US Secret Service and the US Department of Education reviewed all targeted school violence incidents from 1974 to June 2000 and identified behavioral warning signs in 93% of the cases.[69] In 81% of the incidents, other people, often the shooter's peers, had some knowledge of the plans.[69] In a follow-up study conducted from 2008 to 2017, researchers found that 100% of the perpetrators showed concerning behaviors, and in 77% of school shooting incidents at least 1 person knew about the attackers plan.[70] These numbers represent an important place for an intervention, and the Start With Hello campaign could be a first step in getting individuals the support that they need. The age level–appropriate curriculum may be effective in helping students identify possible warning signs of potential future attacks and encourage students to feel comfortable telling an adult or mentor about these warning signs without fear of retribution for themselves or the person they are concerned for.[68]

State and Federal Levels

Red flag laws and extreme risk protection orders

In circumstances where the perpetrator is old enough to own a firearm, data on behavioral warning signs also suggest risk-based firearm removal laws could be an effective tool for prevention. Based on the presumption that a person's risk for violence can fluctuate over time, these laws may prevent a firearm associated tragedy by temporarily removing the firearm from the individual. These laws, often referred to as *red flag laws* or *extreme risk protection orders*, are in effect in 19 states and the District of Columbia as of July 2020.[71] The law is specific to each state, but, in most cases, law enforcement or family members may petition a court to temporarily suspend an individual's right to possess or purchase a firearm. Current research is limited but shows promising evidence of the effectiveness of these state-level risk-based firearm removal policies. Two studies evaluated these laws in Connecticut and Indiana.[72,73] The results were inconclusive for violence prevention but promising for suicide prevention. It is important, however, to recognize that this law would not have prevented the mass shooting at Sandy Hook and other school shootings like Sandy Hook. Most school shootings are perpetrated by minors who often already are unable to legally possess a firearm. As long as firearms are as widely accessible as they are in the United States, the effectiveness of this strategy against preventing school shootings still is unknown. Further research is needed in order to adequately assess the realities of both implementing these orders and their resulting effectiveness in addressing violence prevention.

Gun-free zones

In 1990, one of the most well-known instances of a federal law intended to prevent shootings in schools, the Gun-Free School Zones Act of 1990,[74] was passed. The bill outlawed any individual from knowingly possessing a firearm within 1000 ft from school (public or private) grounds, with some exceptions.[74] According to the National Criminal Justice Reference Service, the penalty for breaking this law is a fine up to $5000 or imprisonment of up to 5 years.[75] This policy has become highly politicized in recent years. Just 3 days after the 2012 school shooting at Sandy Hook Elementary School, editorials began to appear online blaming the shooting on the fact Sandy Hook Elementary School was a gun-free zone.[76] Although proponents of the law believe this helps to keep guns away from schools, opponents of gun-free zones believe that perpetrators may target these areas due to the belief that the victims would not be able to defend themselves because they are unarmed. Despite the controversy, there currently is no peer-reviewed evidence to the effectiveness of gun-free zones.[77]

Child access prevention laws

Given that a majority of school shootings are perpetrated by a minor,[9] Child access prevention (CAP) laws could be an effective policy to prevent school shootings. CAP laws require that a firearm is stored and locked properly so that a child would not be able to access it. In most cases, some tragedy with a child must occur for these policies to be invoked.

The RAND Corporation has determined that there is substantial evidence that CAP laws prevent accidental shootings and suicides (the only policy to achieve a "supportive" rating), and there is some evidence that CAP laws also prevent violent crime.[78] In 2020, 29 states and the District of Columbia have implemented some form of CAP law, although the details can vary greatly by jurisdiction. With variation, 14 states and the

District of Columbia require only that the individual was negligent in storing and locking the firearm.[79] In the other 14 states, however, there is an additional requirement that the individual recklessly endangered their child by not properly locking and storing a firearm in order to be charged. In these states, it must be proved that the individual was aware of the risks but disregarded these dangers in their failure to secure their firearm.[79] The punishments for improper storage (either negligent or reckless) also can vary in these states from a misdemeanor to a felony.[79] Therefore, the effectiveness of these laws depends on the specific state.[80]

Other gun safety laws
The authors choose to focus this discussion on the 3 policies discussed previously—red flag/extreme risk protection orders, gun-free zones, and CAP laws—because they have specific qualities to them that suggest they could directly decrease the frequency of K–12 school shootings. Other gun laws, however, such as limits on magazine size, licensing laws, universal background checks, and a ban on assault weapons, also might be effective in reducing these shootings. Research has suggested that conglomerate measures on the permissiveness of gun laws in a state show that more restrictive gun laws are associated with lower mass shootings,[81] for example. Other research has found that specific policies, such as handgun purchaser licensing laws and bans of large-capacity magazines, are associated with fewer mass shootings.[82] More research is needed, however, to determine if these results would be generalizable to K–12 school shootings.

SUMMARY

K–12 school shootings are exceedingly rare events in the United States, but even a single occurrence that places children and their well-being at-risk is 1 too many. Schools should be spaces where students are safe, supported, and able to engage, thrive, and learn. When a school shooting occurs, the harm extends far beyond those who have been physically injured or killed and can have significant effects that have an impact on the mental health, learning, and emotional well-being of children within the school community. There are several current practices and policies in place with the goal of preventing K–12 school shootings; however, these solutions must account for the well-being and developmental needs of children and ensure they are not harmful in their own ways. For example, research has illustrated that metal detectors in schools have the potential to make students feel less safe,[32–34] and arming teachers could increase anxiety of students and teachers alike.[49] At the same time, there are other school safety efforts (for example, behavioral threat assessments, notification technologies, and emergency preparedness drills and programs, among others), which may be effective in deterring school gun violence. Rigorous research, however, is needed to evaluate the effectiveness of these kinds of tactics independently and, perhaps more importantly, in tandem and as part of a school's larger safety plan.

Additionally, some evidence suggests that investing in the implementation of positive youth development programs, increased access to comprehensive mental health care for children, and/or implementing antibullying and inclusion programs ought to be part of a broader and long-term vision for gun violence prevention. Given the critical role schools play in shaping a child's development, schools have the potential to address early antecedents of violence behavior, and investing in this kind of evidence-based programming for students could be an important component without waiting for new laws to be passed.[83] Lastly, and from a policy perspective, the evidence is clear that the passing of specific laws intended to prevent school shootings and other types of gun violence should be a goal—CAP laws, for example, have been shown to be effective at preventing children from accessing firearms.[78] When taken together, this multilevel approach has enormous potential to effectively prevent school shootings and foster the long-term well-being of children.

CLINICAL CARE POINTS

- Gun violence in K–12 schools is a public health crisis that has an impact not only on the children and school staff who are directly injured and killed in these tragic events but also on all members of the school community who were indirectly exposed to this violence.

- It is estimated that more than 240,000 children have been exposed to gun violence in schools over the past 2 decades, with black children impacted at disproportionately high rates.

- K–12 schools ought to be safe spaces where children can thrive. There are limited data quantifying the short-term and long-term impacts of school shootings on child health and learning outcomes.

- Solutions to the persistence of gun violence in K–12 schools must require a multifaceted and coordinated effort that draws on a wide range of evidence-informed strategies that also consider the well-being of children in their approach.

- There is limited evidence regarding the effectiveness of physical security measures; however, school-wide efforts to address early antecedents of aggressive behaviors in youth and policies that make it harder for youth to have access to guns and promote safe firearm practices collectively could help reduce K–12 school shootings.

DISCLOSURES

The authors have nothing to disclose.

REFERENCES

1. Klarevas L. Rampage nation. Promethus Books; 2016.
2. Vance P. State police identify weapons used in sandy hook investigation; investigation continues. State of Connecticut. Department of Emergency Services and Public Protection; 2013. Available at: https://web.archive.org/web/20160517175905/http://www.ct.gov/despp/cwp/view.asp?A=4226&Q=517284. Accessed July 2020.
3. Shultz JM, Muschert GW, Dingwall A, et al. The sandy hook elementary school shooting as tipping point: "this time is different". Disaster Health 2013;1(2):65–73.
4. Astor M. Newtown wasn't an end for gun control. It was a beginning. New York times 2019. Available at: https://www.nytimes.com/2019/04/29/us/politics/newtown-parkland-guns.html. Accessed July 2020.
5. Booty M, O'Dwyer J, Webster D, et al. Describing a "mass shooting": the role of databases in understanding burden. Inj Epidemiol 2019;6:47.
6. America's Children: Key National Indicators of Well-Being (NA). U.S. Government Printing Office; 2019.
7. Women and children in the crosshairs: new analysis of mass shootings in America reveals 54 percent involved domestic violence and 25 percent of fatalities were children. Everytown for Gun Safety. Published 2017. Available at: https://everytown.org/press/women-and-children-in-the-crosshairs-new-analysis-of-mass-shootings-in-america-reveals-54-percent-involved-domestic-violence-and-25-percent-of-fatalities-were-children/. Accessed July 1, 2020.

8. Levy M, Safcsak K, Dent DL, et al. Mass shootings: are children safer in the streets than in the home? J Pediatr Surg 2019;54(1):150–4.
9. Reeping PM, Klarevas LJ, Rajan S, et al. State firearm laws, gun ownership, and K-12 school shootings: implications for school safety. J Sch Violence 2020. Under Revi.
10. Cox J, Rich S, Chiu A, et al. More than 228, 000 students have experienced gun violence at school since columbine. Washington Post. Published 2020. Available at: https://www.washingtonpost.com/graphics/2018/local/school-shootings-database/. Accessed July 2020.
11. Rajan S, Branas CC, Myers D, et al. Youth exposure to violence involving a gun: evidence for adverse childhood experience classification. J Behav Med 2019; 42(4):646–57.
12. Luthar SS, Goldstein A. Children's exposure to community violence: implications for understanding risk and resilience. J Clin Child Adolesc Psychol 2004;33(3): 499–505.
13. Garbarino J, Bradshaw CP, Vorrasi JA. Mitigating the effects of gun violence on children and youth. Future Child 2002;12(2):73–85.
14. Harding DJ, Fox C, Mehta JD. Studying rare events through qualitative case studies: lessons from a study of rampage school shootings. Sociol Methods Res 2002;31(2):174–217.
15. Kleck G, Kappas J, Goyal MK, et al. School shootings during 2013–2015 in the USA. Aggress Behav 2019;39(1):321–7.
16. Callcut RA, Robles AM, Kornblith LZ, et al. Effect of mass shootings on gun sales - a 20 year perspective. J Trauma Acute Care Surg 2019. https://doi.org/10.1097/TA.0000000000002399.
17. Burns R, Crawford C. School shootings, the media, and public fear: Ingredients-for a moral panic. Crime Law Soc Change 1999;32(2):147–68.
18. Dann C. Mass shootings, economy ranked as most significant news events of 2018. ABC News. Published 2018. Available at: https://www.nbcnews.com/politics/meet-the-press/mass-shootings-economy-ranked-most-significant-news-events-2018-n948201. Accessed July 2020.
19. Van Gerwen LJ, Spinhoven P, Dickstra RFW, et al. People who seek help for fear of flying: typology of flying phobics. Behav Ther 1997;28(2):237–51.
20. Benjet C, Bromet E, Karam EG, et al. The epidemiology of traumatic event exposure worldwide: results from the World mental health survey consortium. Psychol Med 2016;46(2):327–43.
21. Jackson FM, James SA, Owens TC, et al. Erratum to: anticipated negative police-youth encounters and depressive symptoms among pregnant african american women: a brief report. J Urban Health 2017;94(3):457.
22. Pryor DW, Hughes MR. Fear of rape among college women: a social psychological analysis. Violence Vict 2013;28(3):443–65.
23. Cornell DG, Mayer MJ. Why do school order and safety matter? Educ Res 2010; 39(1):7–15.
24. Lowe SR, Galea S. The mental health consequences of mass shootings. Trauma Violence Abuse 2017;18(1):62–82.
25. Stene LE, Schultz J-H, Dyb G. Returning to school after a terror attack: a longitudinal study of school functioning and health in terror-exposed youth. Eur Child Adolesc Psychiatry 2019;28(3):319–28.
26. Teigen KH, Jensen TK. Unlucky victims or lucky survivors?: Spontaneous counterfactual thinking by families exposed to the tsunami disaster. Eur Psychol 2011; 16(1):48–57.

27. Pawlowski A. Parkland, Sandy Hook suicides show lingering trauma. Today 2019. Available at: https://www.today.com/health/understanding-survivor-s-guilt-parkland-sandy-hook-suicides-show-lingering-t150981. Accessed July 2020.

28. Madan M. Leaders react and take steps after second tragedy at Parkland. Miami Herald 2019. Available at: https://www.miamiherald.com/news/local/community/broward/article228350134.html. Accessed July 2020.

29. Warnick BR, Kapa R. Protecting students from gun violence. Does "Target Hardening" do more harm than good? Educ Next 2019;19(2):22–8.

30. Farmer S. Criminality of black youth in inner-city schools: "Moral panic", moral imagination, and moral formation. Race Ethn Educ 2010;13(3):367–81.

31. Zhe EJ, Nickerson AB. Effects of an intruder crisis drill on children's knowledge, anxiety, and perceptions of school safety. School Psych Rev 2007;36(3):501–8.

32. Mowen TJ, Freng A. Is more necessarily better? School security and perceptions of safety among students and parents in the United States. Am J Crim Justice 2019;44(3):376–94.

33. Perumean-Chaney SE, Sutton LM. Students and perceived school safety: the impact of school security measures. Am J Crim Justice 2013;38(4):570–88.

34. Gastic B. Metal detectors and feeling safe at school. Educ Urban Soc 2011;43(4):486–98.

35. Connell NM. Fear of crime at school: understanding student perceptions of safety as function of historical context. Youth Violence Juv Justice 2018;16(2):124–36.

36. Tanner-Smith EE, Fisher BW. Visible school security measures and student academic performance, attendance, and postsecondary aspirations. J Youth Adolesc 2016;45(1):195–210.

37. Cuellar MJ. School safety strategies and their effects on the occurrence of school-based violence in U.S. high schools: an exploratory study. J Sch Violence 2018;17(1):28–45.

38. Graves KN, Frabutt JM, Med DV, et al. Teaching conflict resolution skills to middle and high school students through interactive drama and role play teaching conflict resolution skills to middle and high school students through interactive drama and role play. J Sch Violence 2007;6(4):57–9.

39. Kelly ZV. Establishing a safe school culture: an examination of current practices in K through 12 leadership. Published online 2017. Available at: https://digitalcommons.pepperdine.edu/etd/775/.

40. Borum R, Cornell DG, Modzeleski W, et al. What can be done about school shootings?: a review of the evidence. Educ Res 2010;39(1):27–37.

41. Musu L, Zhang A, Wang K, et al. Indicators of school crime and safety: 2018. Published online 2019. Available at: https://nces.ed.gov/pubsearch/pubsinfo.asp?pubid=2019047.

42. Jonson CL, Moon MM, Hendry JA. One size does not fit all: traditional lockdown versus multioption responses to school shootings. J Sch Violence 2018. https://doi.org/10.1080/15388220.2018.1553719.

43. Blad E. Do schools''active-shooter'drills prepare or frighten? Educ Dig 2018;83(6):4–8.

44. Mazzei P. Parkland gunman carried out rampage without entering a single classroom. New York Times. Published 2018. Available at: https://www.nytimes.com/2018/04/24/us/parkland-shooting-reconstruction.html. Accessed July 2020.

45. Gubiotti M. Opposing viewpoints: preparing students, teachers, and the community for school shootings: saving lives with active shooter simulations. Child Leg Rights J 2015;35(3):254.

46. Waselewski M, Patterson BA, Chang T, et al. Active shooter drills in the United States: a national study of youth experiences and perceptions. J Adolesc Health 2020;67(4):509–13.

47. Rygg L. School shooting simulations: at what point does preparation become more harmful than helpful. Child Leg Rts J 2015;35:215.

48. Erbacher TA, Poland S. School psychologists must be involved in planning and conducting active shooter drills. Communique 2019;48(1):10–2.

49. Rajan S, Branas CC. Arming schoolteachers: what do we know? where do we go from here? Am J Public Health 2018;108(7):860–2.

50. Reaves BA, Trotter AL. The state of law enforcement training academies. Sheriff & Deputy Dated. Published online 2017;44–7.

51. Yacek D. America's armed teachers: an ethical analysis. Teach Coll Rec 2018; 120(8). Available at: https://www.scopus.com/inward/record.uri?eid=2-s2.0-85068428892&partnerID=40&md5=7e15fc2020e74000ab297063e292186c.

52. Brenan M. Most US teachers oppose carrying guns in schools. Gallup. Published 2018. Available at: https://news.gallup.com/poll/229808/teachers-oppose-carrying-guns-schools.aspx. Accessed July 2020.

53. Waldman C. "Is my child safe at school?" new poll captures parents' concerns on school safety, guns for teachers. Alliance for Excellent Education; 2018. Available at: https://all4ed.org/is-my-child-safe-at-school-new-poll-captures-parents-concerns-on-school-safety-guns-for-teachers/. Accessed July 2020.

54. Hill EW. The cost of arming schools: the price of stopping a bad guy with a gun. Urban Publ. Published online 2013. Available at: https://engagedscholarship.csuohio.edu/urban_facpub/678. Accessed July 2020.

55. Lesko N. Act your age!: a cultural construction of adolescence. London: Routledge Farmer; 2001.

56. Collaborative for academic, social, and emotional learning. Casel. Available at: https://casel.org/. Accessed July 2020.

57. Brendtro LK, Long NJ. Violence begets violence: breaking conflict cycles. J Emot Behav Probl 1994;3(1):2–7.

58. Kellam SG, Wang W, Mackenzie ACL, et al. The impact of the good behavior game, a universal classroom-based preventive intervention in first and second grades, on high-risk sexual behaviors and drug abuse and dependence disorders into young adulthood. Prev Sci 2014;15(1):6–18.

59. Kellam SG, Mackenzie ACL, Brown CH, et al. The good behavior game and the future of prevention and treatment. Addict Sci Clin Pract 2011;6(1):73.

60. Oriol X, Miranda R, Amutio A, et al. Violent relationships at the social-ecological level: a multi-mediation model to predict adolescent victimization by peers, bullying and depression in early and late adolescence. PLoS One 2017;12(3): e0174139.

61. Mitchell MM, Bradshaw CP. Examining classroom influences on student perceptions of school climate: the role of classroom management and exclusionary discipline strategies. J Sch Psychol 2013;51(5):599–610.

62. Bradshaw CP, Milam AJ, Furr-Holden CDM, et al. The school assessment for environmental typology (SAfETy): an observational measure of the school environment. Am J Community Psychol 2015;56(3–4):280–92.

63. Shackleton N, Jamal F, Viner RM, et al. School-based interventions going beyond health education to promote adolescent health: systematic review of reviews. J Adolesc Health 2016;58(4):382–96.

64. Melendez-Torres GJ, Dickson K, Fletcher A, et al. Systematic review and meta-analysis of effects of community-delivered positive youth development interventions on violence outcomes. J Epidemiol Community Health 2016;70(12):1171–7.

65. Gonzalez-Guarda RM, Dowdell EB, Marino MA, et al. American academy of nursing on policy: recommendations in response to mass shootings. Nurs Outlook 2018;66(3):333–6.

66. Leary MR, Kowalski RM, Smith L, et al. Teasing, rejection, and violence: case studies of the school shootings. Aggress Behav 2003;29(3):202–14.

67. Landau E. Rejection, bullying are risk factors among shooters. CNN 2012;19:12.

68. Start with Hello. Sandy hook Promise. Available at: https://www.sandyhookpromise.org/our-programs/start-with-hello/. Accessed July 2020.

69. Vossekuil B, Fein RA, Reddy M, et al. The final report and findings of the safe school initiative. Washington, DC: US Secret Serv Dep Educ.; 2002.

70. Alathari L, Drysdale D, Driscoll S, et al. Protecting America's schools: A US Secret Service analysis of targeted school violence. Published online 2019. Available at: https://www.secretservice.gov/sites/default/files/2020-04/Protecting_Americas_Schools.pdf.

71. Extreme risk protection. Giffords law center. Available at: https://lawcenter.giffords.org/gun-laws/policy-areas/who-can-have-a-gun/extreme-risk-protection-orders/. Accessed July 2020.

72. Swanson JW, Easter MM, Alanis-Hirsch K, et al. Criminal justice and suicide outcomes with Indiana's risk-based gun seizure law. J Am Acad Psychiatry Law 2019;47(2):188–97.

73. Swanson JW, Norko MA, Lin H-J, et al. Implementation and effectiveness of Connecticut's risk-based gun removal law: does it prevent suicides. L Contemp Probs 2017;80:179.

74. Gun-free zones act of 1990. US Congress, and the United States of America; 1990. p. 4844–5.

75. Gun-Free Zones Act of 1990. Available at: http://www.ncjrs.gov/App/publications/abstract.aspx?ID=140617%0A. Accessed July 2020.

76. Lesson of sandy hook, clackamas — ban gun-free zones. Available at: https://www.investors.com/politics/editorials/sandy-hook-tragedy-prevented-at-clackamas/. Accessed July 2020.

77. Morral A, Ramchand R, Smart R. The science of gun policy 2018. Available at: http://228.60.152.13/RAND_RR2088.pdf.

78. What science tells us about the effects of gun policies. RAND Corporation. Available at: https://www.rand.org/research/gun-policy/key-findings/what-science-tells-us-about-the-effects-of-gun-policies.html. Accessed July 2020.

79. The effects of child-access prevention laws. RAND corporation. Available at: https://www.rand.org/research/gun-policy/analysis/child-access-prevention.html. Accessed July 2020.

80. Hamilton EC, Miller CC III, Cox CS Jr, et al. Variability of child access prevention laws and pediatric firearm injuries. J Trauma Acute Care Surg 2018;84(4):613–9.

81. Reeping PM, Cerda M, Kalesan B, et al. State gun laws, gun ownership, and mass shootings in the US: cross sectional time series. BMJ 2019;364:l542.

82. Webster DW, McCourt AD, Crifasi CK, et al. Evidence concerning the regulation of firearms design, sale, and carrying on fatal mass shootings in the United States. Criminol Public Policy 2020;19(1):171–212.

83. Branas CC, Reeping PM, Rudolph KE. Beyond gun laws – innovative interventions to reduce gun violence in the United States. JAMA Psychiatry 2020. https://doi.org/10.1001/jamapsychiatry.2020.2493.

Sexual Violence Against Children

Ingrid Walker-Descartes, MD, MPH, MBA[a],*, Gillian Hopgood, DO[a],
Luisa Vaca Condado, BA[a], Lori Legano, MD[b]

KEYWORDS

- Child sexual violence • Commercial sexual exploitation • Child marriages
- Sexual abuse • Female genital mutilation

KEY POINTS

- Sexual violence against children is a crime that has both short- and long-term consequences and interferes with their developmental trajectory and long-term quality of life.
- There is significant overlap in the mental health sequelae for child victims of sexual violence, which includes sex trafficking, sexual abuse, child marriages, and female genital mutilation.
- Continued data and in-depth primary research need to be generated on the different forms of violence against children, particularly in low- and middle-income countries to bolster stronger arguments for effective policy-making.

INTRODUCTION

Sexual violence against children is a gross violation of their rights during their formative years and will likely interfere with their developmental trajectory and long-term quality of life. Children are at risk in their homes, institutions (academic and religious), workplaces, travel and tourism facilities, and their communities.[1] The dualism of technology in its role of maximizing opportunities for exploitation, while having the potential to play a powerful role in its prevention, gives children ready access to sexually explicit content. Adult perpetrators may also have ready access to children. This technological bridge facilitates grooming and the eventual luring of many children who are eventually victimized. The UNICEF study, *Hidden in Plain Sight*, estimated that around 120 million girls under the age of 20 (about 1 in 10) have been exploited through forced sexual intercourse or other forced sexual acts at some point of their lives.[2] Boys also report sexual violence, but to a lesser extent than girls. Although more recent global estimates on sexual violence among boys are unavailable because of the lack of

[a] Department of Medical Education-Pediatrics, Maimonides Children's Hospital of Brooklyn, 4802 Tenth Avenue, Brooklyn, NY 11219, USA; [b] Department of Pediatrics, Bellevue Hospital Center, 462 First Avenue, New York, NY 10016, USA
* Corresponding author.
E-mail address: lwalker-descartes@maimonidesmed.org

Pediatr Clin N Am 68 (2021) 427–436
https://doi.org/10.1016/j.pcl.2020.12.006
0031-3955/21/© 2020 Elsevier Inc. All rights reserved.

comparable data in most countries, girls typically report lifetime rates 3 times higher than boys in high-income countries.[1]

DISCUSSION
Abduction and Trafficking of Children and Adolescents

Commercial sexual exploitation of children (CSEC) is defined as the engagement of any child less than 18 years old in sexual activity in exchange for something of perceived value, such as money, food, or shelter.[3] CSEC has several forms, including sex trafficking, prostitution, sex tourism, pornography, early marriage, performance in sexual venues, and online or electronic transmission of children engaged in sexual activities.[4] As a form of human trafficking, the exploitation of these children can also appear as forced labor, bonded labor, involuntary domestic servitude, child soldier recruitment, and debt bondage among migrant laborers.[5] To ensure compliance, children may be drugged, abducted, or promised a better life.[3] The realization that this is not the case often comes too late.

Having no centralized database to tally the victim impact of this crime, the prevalence of child sex trafficking is difficult to determine. The International Labor Organization estimates that of the more than 1 million victims of forced sexual exploitation, about 21% of all victims were identified as children under 18 years of age.[3] Current prevalence estimates for CSEC in US health care settings (ie, emergency departments, child advocacy centers, and teen clinics) approximate victims to be 11.0% of patients seen in these encounters.[6] Other recent estimates by global organizations suggest that around 24.9 million people worldwide are current victims of human trafficking. The proportion attributable to sex trafficking remains unknown.[7] Considering the challenges to derive CSEC statistics, available research highlights sex trafficking to be most common in Europe, Central Asia, and the Americas.[8]

Intrafamilial Abuse

Intrafamilial child sexual abuse (CSA) as a form of sexual violence remains a global problem. To gain an international perspective, a meta-analysis combined prevalence estimates of CSA reported in 217 publications published between 1980 and 2008. Three hundred thirty-one independent samples were analyzed, with a total of 9,911,748 participants. This study identified a global prevalence rate of 13%. One-third of these reported cases of CSA identified the perpetrator to be a family member, with fathers and stepfathers representing the majority of convicted offenders.[9] Self-reported CSA was more common among female (180/1000) than male participants (76/1000).[7] Disclosure trends are not surprising given societal pressures around manhood and masculinity, making it more palatable for women and girls to disclose their victimization in comparison to their male counterparts.[10] Other contributors to nondisclosure stem from their developmental vulnerability, allowing children who have been manipulated to feel responsible for their abuse.[11] Many caregivers further complicate these feelings, asking children after disclosure, "Why did you allow that to happen?"[12] More significantly, most perpetrators are dominant male figures in the household. The child victim may be concerned about the consequences for the perpetrator. These abusers are familiar figures who develop complex, confusing, and ambivalent relationships with the children they victimize.[13] In some instances, children, fearing that their disclosure will not be believed, or that it will negatively affect their own well-being and that of the family, are then made to endure further abuse with their silence.[12]

CSA cooccurs with other forms of abuse or neglect, especially in family environments, with an interplay of multiple factors that are not unique to CSA. Some of these family demographic factors, as related to CSA, include low family support, high stress attributed to poverty, low parental education, absent or single parenting, parental substance abuse, domestic violence, or an emotionally unavailable caregiver.[13,14] Child-related factors are also at play. Children described as impulsive, emotionally needy, and/or who have learning or physical disabilities, mental health problems, or substance use are at increased risk.[15,16] Out-of-home youth are also particularly vulnerable. This risk to these youths is potentiated initially as a condition that leads to their out-of-home status and later as a consequence of situations stemming from their living on the streets.[17–19] Once on the streets, these youths may be exploited and forced to trade sex for survival needs, such as food, shelter, money, or drugs.[19–21] In many countries, where children living on the streets are in conflict with the law, there is an additional risk of sexual violence by authorities on the street and in facilities where these children are detained.[22]

Child Marriage

Child marriage involves the formal or informal union of a child under the age of 18 with another child or an adult.[23] This event is recognized by the United Nations Populations Fund (UNFPA) as a human rights violation along the continuum of sexual violence against children.[23–25] Although the global prevalence of the practice has decreased by 15% in the last decade, the practice remains a significant problem worldwide.[23] According to the United Nations Children's Fund (UNICEF), this systemic form of gender-based violence impacts more than 700 million women alive today who were married before the age of 18.[23] Ingrained societal norms around traditional customs and religious beliefs of gender roles further support the practice.[23–25] Data provided by UNFPA estimate that 1 in 3 girls globally are married before age 18.[23] Although boys are likewise impacted by the practice, girls are overwhelmingly more affected, with prevalence estimates of affected boys to be about one/sixth that of affected girls.[25]

At its core, child marriage is a function of poverty. Children living in the world's lowest income countries are most susceptible to forced early marriage, whereby many families may marry off their children as a commercial exchange or for perceived opportunity.[26] South Asia has the highest prevalence of child marriage (42%), with India accounting for one-third of the global total. The 10 highest prevalence countries are concentrated in South Asia and sub-Saharan Africa. Nigeria has the highest overall prevalence of child marriage globally, whereas Bangladesh displays the highest rate of girls married before the age of 15.[23]

The consequences of early marriage are grave for the developing children and their futures. Cessation of education and poor health outcomes, especially reproductive health, are among the major disadvantages of this decision.[26–29] Because of lower levels of awareness and knowledge about sexually transmitted diseases, an apparent paradox characterizes the impact of HIV/AIDS on child marriages in affected countries. Instead of serving as a protective factor, ironically, marriage appears to expose rather than shield young women because of an often violent transition from virginity to frequent episodes of forced, unprotected sex.[29] These negative consequences continue to compound with pregnancy with poor birth outcomes. Early motherhood challenges the body's ability to accommodate a pregnancy during a time of intense growth spurts. The body's competing physiologic priorities result in an aggravated state of malnutrition. As malnutrition operates as a chronic medical condition with associated morbidities, these malnourished young mothers are prone to delivering low-birth-weight babies susceptible to this same chronic condition.[30] As a result, complications during pregnancy and childbirth not only are risky for the mother but also can lead to the death of the child. Evidence shows that young maternal age at birth, short interpregnancy intervals, and poor access to adequate prenatal care are core determinants of infant deaths among births to young mothers.[30] With these realities, encouraging a postponement of the physiologic time for childbearing, in situations of limited access to reproductive and sexual health information and services, appears a practical approach to mitigate the situations resulting in large family size and increased burden on these girls.[23]

Strategies to end the practice of child marriage include both global campaigns and grassroots programs focused on mitigating poverty through education and work opportunities for children and their communities.[25] Legislative efforts to outlaw the practice have also been successful at decreasing the rate of formal child marriages. With acceleration of these efforts worldwide, the United Nations Sustainable Development Goals have called for an end to child marriage by the year 2030.[28]

Female Genital Mutilation

Female genital mutilation (FGM) is defined by the World Health Organization (WHO) and the United Nations agencies as "the partial or total removal of the female external genitalia or other injury to the female genital organs for non-medical reasons."[31,32] There are 4 classifications based on the nature of the disfigurement:

- Type I: the partial or total removal of the clitoral glans (the external and visible part of the clitoris, which is a sensitive part of the female genitals) and/or the prepuce/clitoral hood (the fold of skin surrounding the clitoral glans)[33]
- Type II: the partial or total removal of the clitoral glans and the labia minora (the inner folds of the vulva), with or without removal of the labia majora (the outer folds of skin of the vulva)[33]
- Type III: the narrowing of the vaginal opening through the creation of a covering seal formed by cutting and repositioning the labia minora, or labia majora, or sometimes through stitching, with or without removal of the clitoral prepuce/clitoral hood and glans (type I FGM) (also known as infibulation)[33]
- Type IV: all other harmful procedures to the female genitalia for nonmedical purposes, for example, pricking, piercing, incising, scraping, and cauterizing the genital area[33]

Defibulation, the reversal of infibulation, is the practice of cutting open the sealed vaginal opening of a women to allow intercourse or to facilitate childbirth and is often necessary for improving health and well-being of these victims.[33]

In line with its classification as a harmful practice, FGM is said to violate the human rights of girls and women on par with child marriage by the Convention on the Elimination of all Forms of Discrimination against Women and the Committee on the Rights of the Child Committee.[34] Despite this classification, this practice remains a deeply rooted tradition in many communities in Africa, Asia, and the Middle East. FGM continues to be another form of sexual violence enforced as a traditional custom performed on young girls some time between infancy and age 15 in preparation for marriage.[30,35] In several cultures, female circumcision is perpetuated as a rite of passage. Girls are forced to endure this event as a violent initiation into other forms of sexual control they are expected to undergo for the rest of their lives, in particular, after achieving puberty and entering marriage.[35]

Like all invasive procedures, FGM is not without short-term consequences and long-term health risks. Every type of FMG is associated with a series of long-term health risks.[32] The most common short-term consequences of FGM include shock secondary to excessive bleeding (hemorrhage) or severe pain owing to swelling, causing difficulty in passing urine and feces, or from infections.[32,33] In worst case scenarios, death ensues from complications from hemorrhaging or infections (ie, tetanus).[33] Abscesses and dermoid cysts are common complications, leading to chronic pelvic infections and chronic pain (ie, back and pelvic pain), urinary problems (ie, urinary tract infections or painful urination), and menstrual problems (ie, painful menstruation, difficulty passing menstrual blood).[32,33] WHO-led studies on FGM further validates the association of birth complications for both mother and child being commensurate with the severity of disfigurement from FMG. Rates of cesarean section and postpartum hemorrhage were both more frequent in women with FGM compared with those who did not experience FGM. Rates of caesarean section showed a 29% increase for type II and 31% increase for type III FGM. Postpartum hemorrhage showed a 21% increase for type II and 69% for type III FGM among women with FGM compared with those without FGM. There was also an increased probability of tearing and recourse to episiotomies, while specific risks to the infant of a mother who had experienced FGM showed significantly higher death rates (including stillbirths). There was a 15% increase in stillbirths for type I FGM, a 32% increase for type II FGM, and 55% increase for type III FGM.[32]

In 2013, UNICEF estimated that more than 125 million girls and women have been cut in the 29 countries in Africa and the Middle East, where FGM is concentrated.[35] An additional 30 million girls were projected to be at risk of being cut over the next decade if trends are not reversed by current interventions.[36] In their most recent update, UNICEF notes the practice has changed in several ways, including a noticeable decline in some countries. This decline was demonstrated with a review of demographic health surveys comparing the incidence of the practice in the cohorts of women in 45 to 49 age group versus the 15 to 19 age group. The 15 to 19 age group reported that a noticeable proportion of them had not experienced this procedure.[33]

The Impact of Sexual Violence Against Children

Evidence shows that sexual violence can have serious short- and long-term physical, psychological, and social consequences for girls, boys, their families, and their communities. The impact of this form of violence on the mental health in trafficked children remains complex, having both physical and psychological consequences. The consequences to their physical health are unwanted pregnancy, sexually transmitted infections, substance use, and traumatic injury.[1] The psychological consequences, which may include posttraumatic stress disorder, depression, anxiety, and behavioral problems, contribute to the resultant decline in lifetime acheivement.[1,2] To contextualize some of these complex dynamics, a study of trafficked children accessing emergency medical services in the United States identified 38.5% of these children having a history of mental disorder, although it is unclear what proportion of their symptoms preceded versus followed their trafficking experience.[37]

Dynamics around the impact of child marriages, mired with cultural underpinnings, remains no less convoluted. Although there has been growing interest in the consequences of child marriage on physical health, the focus of its impact on the psychological well-being of young spouses has been less represented in the literature. An investigation into the effects of sexual violence against children in early marriage requires due attention paid to the trauma that physical and psychological abuse compounded by exploitation may cause.[38] When the body and the mind of a child have not yet reached cognitive and sexual maturity, systematic abuse in the sexual sphere, aggravated by isolation and other forms of violence, not only severely impacts physical well-being but also poses serious mental health challenges.[38] It has been found that these married girls exhibit a similar symptomatic profile of CSA victims with severe signs of posttraumatic stress.[39,40] During the formative years, an event like marriage significantly hampers the balanced psychological, emotional, and social development of a child. To emerge as a psychologically intact adult who is truly ready to embrace the responsibilities of such an arrangement, a child needs an appropriately supported experience of adolescence.[39] This experience will be less likely to occur if the child is forced into an early marriage.

Along the continuum of sexual violence against children, childhood sexual abuse has been associated with increased risk for a multitude of acute and long-term psychological and physical health problems. Comorbidities include depression, posttraumatic stress, and substance abuse problems, as well as sexual revictimization in adolescence and adulthood.[40–42] These psychological effects may manifest differently depending on the age of the child, whereby younger children may act out, develop a decline in their academic performance, or appear anxious or sad; whereas adolescents may exhibit depression, anxiety, low self-esteem, higher rates of self-harm, especially with an early age of onset of their abuse as well as prematurely experiencing their consensual sexual debut and greater number of sexual partners.[43,44] Research consistently demonstrates that certain risk factors increase the severity of childhood sexual abuse–related sequelae, such as abuse that involves penetration, greater frequency, longer duration, use of force, a closer relationship between the child and the perpetrator, physical injury during the abuse, and a lack of caregiver support.[42] Conversely, certain protective factors, such as a child's coping strategies and the availability of stable, supportive caregivers, can ameliorate the adverse impact of childhood sexual abuse, mitigating the late sequelae of CSA seen in victimized adults who disproportionately use health care services and incur greater health care costs compared with adults who did not experience this type of abuse.[45,46]

The mental health sequelae associated with FGM are often downplayed in comparison to the obstetric and gynecologic complications. These documented negative psychological effects include posttraumatic stress disorder, anxiety, depression, and psychosexual problems. A recent study shows that women who have undergone FGM may be more likely than others to experience psychological disturbances (psychiatric diagnosis, anxiety, somatization, phobia, and low self-esteem).[47,48] Based on the type of disfigurement, many report the recollection of the event serves as a paralyzing vivid memory whereby the predominant coping style is avoidance often through substance abuse.[48] Women who have undergone FGM may also be affected by chronic pain syndrome. As with other causes of chronic pain, there is an increased risk of depressed mood, feelings of worthlessness, guilt, and even suicidal ideation. In addition, limited mobility also leads to reduced social functioning and an increased sense of isolation for these women.[49]

SUMMARY

Violence against children inflicts damage at the individual, family, community, and societal level, including direct and indirect costs from increased social spending and lost economic productivity. A study highlighted by UNICEF estimates that the global economic impacts and costs resulting from the consequences of physical, psychological, and sexual violence against children can be as high as $7 trillion.[50] In comparison, this massive cost is thought to be higher than the investment required to prevent much of that violence.[50] The evidence shows that prevention is worth the investment, but prioritizing this agenda to ensure funding through government spending on preventive and responsive actions in relation to violence against children remains very low. Despite funding realities, research and advocacy efforts must continue, with a focus on promoting effective practices for prevention while striving to ensure funding will be prioritized on the global agenda. Continued data and in-depth primary research need to be generated regarding the different forms of violence against children, particularly in low- and middle-income countries. Calculating and reporting theses economic costs often bolster stronger arguments for effective policy-making; however, we cannot lose sight of the importance of the 4 core principles of the rights of children as outlined by the United Nations Convention on the Rights of the Child. On the individual, family, community, and societal level, we must prioritize the rights of children to live free of discrimination, live in households, communities, and a society that remain devoted to the best interests of the child, while ensuring that all children have the right to life, survival, and development.[50,51]

CLINICS CARE POINTS

- Sexual violence is a crime against children that interferes with their developmental trajectory and long-term quality of life. Optimized secondary preventative efforts require the coordinated efforts of health care providers, child welfare agencies, and the court system for tailored treatment and rehabilitative services.

- Children are developmentally vulnerable and are often manipulated to feel guilty or responsible for their abuse, leading to deceased rates of disclosure.

- Lower levels of awareness and knowledge about sexually transmitted diseases derive an apparent paradox for the impact of HIV/AIDS on early marriages, as it is a risk factor and not a protective factor for exposure to the virus for child brides.

- Studies on female genital mutilation strengthens the association between this invasive nonmedical procedure and the increased risk for complications for both mother and child during childbirth.

- There is significant overlap in the mental health consequences of all forms of sexual violence against children, with married girls exhibiting a similar symptomatic profile as child sexual abuse victims.

DISCLOSURE

The authors have nothing to disclose.

REFERENCES

1. United Nations Children's Fund. Sexual violence against children. 2018. Available at: https://www.unicef.org/protection/57929_58006.html. Accessed August 5, 2020.
2. United Nations Children's Fund. Hidden in plain sight: a statistical analysis of violence against children. New York: UNICEF; 2014.
3. Greenbaum J. Child sex trafficking and commercial sexual exploitation. Adv Pediatr 2018;65(1):55–70.
4. Office of Juvenile Justice and Delinquency Prevention (OJJDP). Commercial sexual exploitation of children. Available at: https://ojjdp.ojp.gov/programs/commercial-sexual-exploitation-children. Accessed August 5, 2020.
5. U.S. Department of State. Trafficking in persons report 2020. Washington, DC: U.S. Department of State; 2020. Available at: https://www.state.gov/wp-content/uploads/2020/06/2020-TIP-Report-Complete-062420-FINAL.pdf. Accessed August 5, 2020.

6. International Labour Office. Global estimates of modern slavery: forced labour and forced marriage. 2017. Available at: https://www.ilo.org/wcmsp5/groups/public/@dgreports/@dcomm/documents/publication/wcms_575479.pdf.   Accessed July 24, 2020.

7. U.S. Department of State. Trafficked in persons report 2019. Washington, DC: U.S. Department of State; 2019. Available at: https://www.state.gov/wp-content/uploads/2019/06/2019-Trafficking-in-Persons-Report.pdf. Accessed August 5, 2020.

8. Greenbaum J. Child sex trafficking and commercial sexual exploitation. Presented at the Annual NCJFCJ Conference. July 15, 2014, Chicago, IL.

9. Ottisova L, Hemmings S, Howard LM, et al. Prevalence and risk of violence and the mental, physical and sexual health problems associated with human trafficking: an updated systematic review. Epidemiol Psychiatr Sci 2016;25(4): 317–41.

10. Easton SD, Saltzman LY, Willis DG. "Would you tell under circumstances like that?": barriers to disclosure of child sexual abuse for men. Psychol Men Masc 2014;15(4):460–9.

11. Varma S, Gillespie S, McCracken C, et al. Characteristics of child commercial sexual exploitation and sex trafficking victims presenting for medical care in the United States. Child Abuse Negl 2015;44:98–105.

12. Walker-Descartes I, Sealy YM, Laraque D, et al. Caregiver perceptions of sexual abuse and its effect on management after a disclosure. Child Abuse Negl 2011; 35(6):437–47.

13. Stoltenborgh M, van Ijzendoorn HM, Euser EM, et al. A global perspective on child sexual abuse: meta-analysis of prevalence around the world. Child Maltreat 2011;16(2):79–101.

14. Paine ML, Hansen DJ. Factors influencing children to self-disclose sexual abuse. Clin Psychol Rev 2002;22:271–95.

15. Perez-Fuentes G, Olfson M, Villegas L, et al. Prevalence and correlates of child sexual abuse: a national study. Compr Psychiatry 2013;54(1):16–27.

16. Butler AC. Child sexual assault: risk factors for girls. Child Abuse Negl 2013; 37(9):643–52.

17. Davies EA, Jones AC. Risk factors in child sexual abuse. J Forensic Leg Med 2013;20(3):146–50.

18. Tyler KA, Hoyt DR, Whitbeck LB, et al. The impact of childhood sexual abuse on later sexual victimization among runaway youth. J Res Adolesc 2001;11(2): 151–76.

19. Stewart AJ, Steiman M, Cauce AM, et al. Victimization and posttraumatic stress disorder among homeless adolescents. J Am Acad Child Adolesc Psychiatry 2004;43(3):325–31.

20. Rew L, Taylor-Seehafer M, Fitzgerald ML. Sexual abuse, alcohol and other drug use, and suicidal behaviors in homeless adolescents. Issues Compr Pediatr Nurs 2001;24(4):225–40.

21. Tyler KA, Johnson KA. Trading sex: voluntary or coerced? The experiences of homeless youth. J Sex Res 2006;43(3):208–16.

22. Wernham M. An outside chance: street children and juvenile justice, an international perspective. London: Consortium of Street Children; 2004. Available at: http://createsolutions.org/docs/resources/Outside%20Chance/PART%201.pdf. Accessed August 5, 2020.

23. United Nations Children's Fund. Child marriage. 2020. Available at: https://www.unicef.org/protection/child-marriage. Accessed July 19, 2020.

24. United Nations Population Fund. Child marriage. 2020. Available at: https://www. unfpa.org/child-marriage. Accessed July 15, 2020.

25. United Nations Population Fund. Marrying too young: end child marriage. 2012. Available at: https://www.unfpa.org/sites/default/files/pub-pdf/MarryingTooYoung. pdf. Accessed August 5, 2020.

26. Riggio Chaudhuri E. Thematic report: unrecognised sexual abuse and exploitation of children in child, early and forced marriage. Ratchathewi (Bangkok): EC-PAT International, Plan International. 2015. Available at: https://www.ecpat.org/wp-content/uploads/2016/04/Child%20Marriage_ENG.pdf. Accessed August 5, 2020.

27. Selby D, Singer C. Child marriage: what you need to know and how you can help end it. 2019. Available at: https://www.globalcitizen.org/en/content/child-marriage-brides-india-niger-syria/. Accessed July 21, 2020.

28. United Nations Children's Fund. Ending child marriage: progress and prospects. New York: UNICEF; 2014. Available at: https://www.unicef.org/media/files/Child_Marriage_Report_7_17_LR..pdf. Accessed August 5, 2020.

29. International Planned Parenthood Federation and the Forum on Marriage and the Rights of Women and Girls. Ending child marriage: a guide or global policy action. London: IPPF; 2007. p. 12. Available at: https://www.ippf.org/sites/default/files/ending_child_marriage.pdf. Accessed August 5, 2020.

30. Raj A, McDougal L, Rusch M. Effects of young maternal age and short interpregnancy interval on infant mortality in south asia. Int J Gynaecol Obstet 2014; 124(1):86–7.

31. World Health Organization. An update on WHO's work on female genital mutilation: progress report. 2011. Available at: https://apps.who.int/iris/bitstream/handle/10665/70638/WHO_RHR_11.18_eng.pdf; jsessionid=DABFBCEB026856A23790D2A7A654E1E2?sequence=1. Accessed August 3, 2020.

32. WHO Study Group on Female Genital Mutilation and Obstetric Outcome, Banks E, Meirek O, et al. Female genital mutilation and obstetric outcome: WHO collaborative prospective study in six African countries. Lancet 2006; 67(9525):1835–41.

33. World Health Organization. Female genital mutilation: key facts. 2020. Available at: https://www.who.int/news-room/fact-sheets/detail/female-genital-mutilation. Accessed August 4, 2020.

34. Committee on the Elimination of Discrimination against Women, Committee on the Rights of the Child. Joint General Recommendation no. 31 of the Committee on the Elimination of Discrimination Against Women/General Comment no. 18 of the Committee on the Rights of the Child on Harmful Practices. 2014. Available at: https://documents.ddsny.un.org/doc/UNDOC/GEN/N14/627/78/PDF/N1462778.pdf?OpenElement. Accessed August 5, 2020.

35. Pankhurst A. Child marriage and female circumcision: evidence from Ethiopia. In: Young Lives Policy Brief 21. 2014. Available at: https://www.younglives.org.uk/sites/www.younglives.org.uk/files/YL-PolicyBrief-21_Child%20Marriage%20and%20FGM%20in%20Ethiopia.pdf. Accessed August 3, 2020.

36. United Nations Children's Fund. Female genital mutilation/cutting: a statistical overview and exploration of the dynamics of change. New York: UNICEF; 2013.

37. Greenbaum VJ, Livings MS, Lai BS, et al. Evaluation of a tool to identify child sex trafficking victims in multiple healthcare settings. J Adolesc Health 2018;63(6): 745–52.

38. International Center for Research on Women. Child marriage and domestic violence. 2007. Available at: https://www.icrw.org/files/images/Child-Marriage-Fact-Sheet-Domestic-Violence.pdf. Accessed August 1, 2020.

39. Sanlaap. Underage marriage in rural west Bengal: a survey based study. Available at: https://childhub.org/en/system/tdf/library/attachments/underage_oct07.pdf?file=1&type=node&id=17974. Accessed August 3, 2020.

40. Cutajar MC, Mullen PE, Ogloff JR, et al. Psychopathology in a large cohort of sexually abused children followed up to 43 years. Child Abuse Negl 2010; 34(11):813–22, 13.

41. Dube SR, Anda RF, Whitfield CL, et al. Long-term consequences of childhood sexual abuse by gender of victim. Am J Prev Med 2005;28(5):430–8.

42. Chiesa A, Goldson E. Child sexual abuse. Pediatr Rev 2017;38(3):105–18.

43. Kendall-Tackett KA, Williams LM, Finkelhor D. Impact of sexual abuse on children: a review and synthesis of recent empirical studies. Psychol Bull 1993; 113(1):164–80.

44. Lopez-Castroman J, Melhem N, Birmaher B, et al. Early childhood sexual abuse increases suicidal intent. World Psychiatry 2013;12(2):149–54.

45. Afifi TO, Macmillan HL. Resilience following child maltreatment: a review of protective factors. Can J Psychiatry 2011;56(5):266–72.

46. Leserman J. Sexual abuse history: prevalence, health effects, mediators, and psychological treatment. Psychosom Med 2005;67:906–15.

47. Berg RC, Denison E, Fretheim A. Psychological, social and sexual consequences of female genital mutilation/cutting (FGM/C): a systematic review of quantitative studies. Oslo (Norway): Knowledge Centre for the Health Services at the Norwegian Institute of Public Health; 2010.

48. Knipscheer J, Vloeberghs E, van der Kwaak A, et al. Mental health problems associated with female genital mutilation. Bjpsych Bull 2015;39(6):273–7.

49. Whitehorn J, Ayonrinde O, Maingay S. Female genital mutilation: cultural and psychological implications. Sexual and Relationship Therapy 2002;17(2):161–70.

50. Pereznieto P, Montes A, Routier S, et al. The cost and economic impact of violence against children. 2014. Available at: https://www.odi.org/sites/odi.org.uk/files/odi-assets/publications-opinion-files/9177.pdf. Accessed August 5, 2020.

51. United Nations Committee on the Rights of the Child. UN general assembly, convention on the rights of the child. 1989, United Nations, Treaty Series, vol. 1577. p. 3. United Nations Human Rights Office of the High Commissioner. Available at: https://www.refworld.org/docid/3ae6b38f0.html. Accessed November 7, 2020.

Use of Children as Soldiers

Ruth A. Etzel, MD, PhD

KEYWORDS

- Mycotoxin • Mental health • Child soldier • Youth soldier
- Post-traumatic stress disorder • War • Conflict • Paris commitments

KEY POINTS

- Children may be used in conflicts as fighters, cooks, porters, messengers, or spies, or for sexual purposes.
- Complex consequences on both physical and mental health are reported among child soldiers.
- One-third to one-half of these children may have clinically significant symptoms of post-traumatic stress disorder.
- The United Nations identified more than 25,000 grave violations against children during armed conflicts in 2019.
- The recruitment and use of children in armed conflicts must stop.

Whether they are playing video games, watching television, or downloading feature length films, children are bombarded on a daily basis with glorified images of guns, battles, and war. Because of their developmental stage, children cannot yet rationally evaluate the pros and cons of personally engaging in war. They may, in fact, see it as an exciting adventure. Recall in *The Red Badge of Courage* how the teenaged soldier in the Civil War thought that going to war would make him a man.

There are numerous reasons why children may be pushed into becoming child soldiers, including poverty, hunger, tribalism, the need to seek refuge, mistreatment at home by the police or other armed groups, or the desire to seek vengeance.[1] They may also be pulled into soldiering to protect themselves from harm[1] or they may even find war compelling. The American propensity to romanticize guns is 1 reason that going to war may attract children. Another reason that youth may be easily recruited as soldiers is that their brains are not fully developed until they reach their early 20s. Children are, at this stage of development, "pliable, exploitable, effective and expendable."[2] **Table 1** shows the stages of adolescence and the changes in brain development at each stage.[3]

Department of Environmental and Occupational Health, Milken Institute School of Public Health, The George Washington University, 950 New Hampshire Avenue, Northwest, Washington, DC 20052, USA
E-mail address: RETZEL@GWU.EDU

Pediatr Clin N Am 68 (2021) 437–447
https://doi.org/10.1016/j.pcl.2020.12.010
pediatric.theclinics.com
0031-3955/21/© 2021 Elsevier Inc. All rights reserved.

Table 1 Development of the adolescent brain	
Age (Stage)	**Characteristics**
Early adolescence (age 10–13 y)	Puberty heightens emotional arousability, sensation seeking, reward orientation
Middle adolescence (age 14–16 y)	Period of heightened vulnerability to risk-taking and problems in regulation of affect and behavior
Late adolescence (age ≥17 years)	Maturation of frontal lobes facilitates regulatory competence

Adapted from Steinberg L. Cognitive and affective development in adolescence. Trends Cogn Sci 2005:9;69–74; with permission.

This lack of full development of the frontal lobes may lead some teenagers to engage in risky behaviors. To illustrate the thoughts of an adolescent, consider the words of a 19-year-old German soldier named Ernst Junger in the first World War:

We had bonded together into one large and enthusiastic group. We shared a yearning for danger, for the experience of the extraordinary. We were enraptured by war. We had set out in a rain of flowers, in a drunken atmosphere of blood and roses. Surely the war had to supply us with what we wanted; the great, the overwhelming, the hallowed experience. We thought of it as manly, as action, a merry dwelling party on flowered, blood-bedewed meadows.[4]

Many soldiers who died in World War I were still in their teens. Junger reports that many of the Germans who fought at Ypres (France) were teenagers, boys fresh from school. Unprepared for the carnage that awaited them, some of them arrived to fight in their school caps. "They were mowed down in the thousands by British rifles and machine guns," records Russell Freedman, "in what became known in Germany as the Kindermord bei Ypern, literally 'the Murder of the Children at Ypres.'"[5]

HEALTH CONSEQUENCES

Military service during adolescence has complex consequences on both physical and mental health. In the UK, Abu-Hayyeh and Singh reviewed the consequences and argued that children should not be recruited as soldiers[6] (**Table 2**). Note that the UK is one of only a handful of countries to recruit 16-year-olds into the armed forces. In March 2018, the UK recruited 2290 youth less than 18 years of age, making up 21% of all the country's army recruits.[6]

PSYCHOLOGICAL WELL-BEING OF CHILD SOLDIERS

In the early twentieth century, it was assumed that the experience of being a child soldier inevitably led to psychological distress. Hilton, acclaimed author of *Lost Horizon*, stated "You can't subject a mere boy to 3 years of intense physical and emotional stress without tearing something to tatters. People would say, I suppose, that he came through without a scratch. But the scratches were there – on the inside."[15]

A study by Slone and Mann[16] of children 0 to 6 years old showed that effects include post-traumatic stress disorder (PTSD) and post-traumatic stress symptoms, behavioral and emotional symptoms, sleep problems, disturbed play, and psychosomatic symptoms. Betancourt and associates[17] reviewed the effects by the gender of the child soldiers. It is now better understood that several factors influence children's

Table 2
Child health in armed conflict

Mechanism	Effect
Mortality	The fatality rate of frontline combat infantry in Afghanistan was 7 times higher than that in the rest of the armed forces.[7]
Illness	Conditions for maintenance of child health deteriorate in war—nutrition, water, safety, sanitation, housing and access to health services. Sustained deficiencies in these areas have been shown to have significant impacts on growth in children and adolescents.[8]
Mental health	Younger military personnel are at greater risk of mental health disorders than their civilian counterparts. Exposure to combat is a risk factor for PTSD and other mental disorders, particularly among younger personnel and individuals with preexisting psychosocial vulnerabilities and mental health conditions.[9] Self-harm and suicides in the UK armed forces are more common among younger personnel and exceed rates for young civilians.[10,11] Rates of alcohol misuse are considerably higher in the UK armed forces than in the general population. Young age is particularly associated with alcohol misuse in the UK armed forces.[12] These problems are related to the isolation and enculturation into military life, the trauma of combat, but also to the higher prevalence of preservice vulnerabilities among young recruits to the armed forces.
Educational outcomes	In the armed forces, educational underachievement is a marked factor for PTSD as well as other common mental disorders, alcohol misuse, aggressive behavior and violence.[13] For instance, one study found a PTSD rate of 8.4% among Iraq War veterans who had joined the armed force with no GCSE qualifications, compared with 3.3% among those with A levels.[14]

Abbreviations: GCSE, General Certificate of Secondary Education; PTSD, post-traumatic stress disorder.
From Abu-Hayyeh R, Singh G. Adverse health effects of recruiting child soldiers. BMJ Paediatr Open. 2019 Feb 25;3(1):e000325; with permission.

well-being, including emotional connections within their families, shared values with the armed group, their bond with the community, and the social–emotional–economic capital available to the child to manage his or her postwar life.[18] In Nepal, on-going structural violence seemed to be more significant in affecting the child soldiers' psychological well-being than the war experience itself.[18] Kizilhan and Noll-Husson[19] found that 48% of former Islamic child soldiers in northern Iraq had PTSD, 46% had depressive symptoms, and 51% had somatic disturbances. This figure was significantly higher than among 2 control groups of boys who were not child soldiers.[19] Both Williams[20] and Fisher and associates[21] reviewed studies of the psychological consequences for children who were exposed to war and natural disasters. One-third to one-half of children affected by armed conflict had clinically significant PTSD symptoms.[21] Whether the PTSD construct is appropriate for use in low- and middle-income countries is not known; the construct developed in high-income Anglophone settings.[21]

TOXIC EXPOSURES

In addition to the psychological hazards, child soldiers may be exposed to a variety of toxic agents in the theater of war. Depending on their age and developmental stage, they may have an increased vulnerability to some agents. Children may be especially susceptible to the effects of exposures to toxic compounds because of their anatomic and physiologic differences from adults and their behaviors (**Table 3**).[22] Compared with adults, children have an increased surface area-to-volume ratio, higher minute ventilation, and breathing zones that are closer to the ground (where compounds that are heavier than air may settle)[22–24] and they may be at higher risk of exposure to and absorption of some chemical and biological agents.[25,26] Children have a greater susceptibility to dehydration and shock from exposure to toxic agents.[24] In addition, their developmental abilities and cognitive levels may impede their ability to escape danger.[23] Children have unique psychological needs and vulnerabilities.[22–24]

Multiple reports have documented the long-term health effects of wartime exposures.[27,28] Child soldiers are often injured by unexploded ordnance (bombs, grenades, and mortar shells) and landmines,[29] sometimes resulting in death or disability. Studies of pregnant women have documented that exposures to chromium and uranium are associated with problematic emotional development among their infants.[30]

Children engaged in war may also suffer from exposure to physical agents such as excess noise:

> My son, five-year-old Heraab, finds himself in a community where he is constantly exposed to the sounds of explosions, smell of smoke, accompanied by the regular shrieking of sirens, be it police or ambulance, or the persistent honking of cars and motorbikes rushing the injured to hospital. He shudders and wakes up at night if a truck passes by with speed, sometimes shaking the windows of our house, thinking it must be another attack. (UNICEF worker in Afghanistan)[31]

WARS IN 2020

Twentieth-century wars were characterized by massive, worldwide conflicts. At the beginning the twenty-first century, that was no longer the case. Most wars were civil wars or conflicts (**Fig. 1**).[32,33] Children were swept up in them, just as they were during

Table 3	
Factors enhancing children's vulnerability to biological agents	
Factors	**Relevant Agents**
Anatomic and physiologic differences • Increased ratio of surface area-to-volume • Higher minute ventilation • Breathing air closer to ground	• T-2 mycotoxins • All aerosolized agents • Denser aerosolized agents
Unique susceptibility/severity	• Smallpox, T-2 mycotoxins, VEE
Developmental considerations • Depending on others for care, more likely to lack knowledge or independent means to seek care or identify and avoid danger	• All agents

Abbreviation: VEE, Venezuelan equine encephalitis.
From Cieslak TJ, Henretig FM. Bioterrorism. Pediatr Ann. 2003;32(3):154–165; with permission.

The World at War in 2020

Countries with reported armed clashes between
state forces and/or rebels in 2020[a]

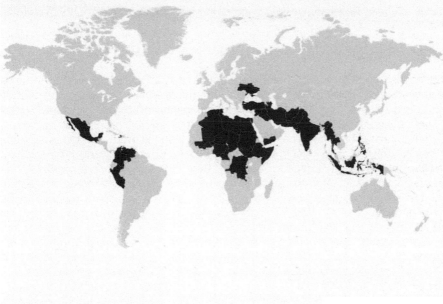

Fig. 1. Countries with armed clashes involving state forces and/or rebel groups in 2020. [a]As of May 2.

earlier, much different twentieth-century wars. **Fig. 1** is based on extensive data collection by the Armed Conflict Location & Event Data Project[32] and shows countries in which there have been reports of armed clashes involving state forces and/or rebel groups in 2020. Even using this simplified definition, the presence of war across the world is extensive.

The issue of child soldiers was hardly a focus of attention during times when child labor was commonplace around the world. It was not until the 1990s that it received attention. In 1996 Ms. Graça Machel, a former Minister of Education of the Republic of Mozambique, gave a groundbreaking report to the United Nations General Assembly on the impact of armed conflict on children. That report put child soldiers in the spotlight.[34] For the first time in history, Machel comprehensively assessed the multiple ways children were abused and brutalized in armed conflicts. The report and a subsequent book[35] called for better protection for children affected by armed conflict. "It is unforgivable that children are assaulted, violated, murdered and yet our conscience is not revolted nor our sense of dignity challenged. This represents a fundamental crisis of our civilization" (Graça Machel).[34]

In this article, the term "child associated with an armed force or armed group" is used synonymously with "child soldier." This is any person younger than 18 years of age who is or who has been recruited or used by an armed force or armed group in any capacity, including but not limited to children, boys and girls, used as fighters, cooks, porters, messengers, spies or for sexual purposes. Previous reports estimated that there were about 250,000 child soldiers in the early 2000s.[36–39] Nearly one-third were girls. Girls may be raped and become pregnant, they may have complications during childbirth, and they may find that their babies are rejected when they return to their villages.[2] **Box 1** shows the countries in which child soldiers are being recruited and used.[40]

GRAVE VIOLATIONS AGAINST CHILDREN

The Machel report prompted the establishment of The Office of the Special Representative of the Secretary-General for Children and Armed Conflict. Subsequently, the United Nations Secretary-General in 2005 identified 6 grave violations against children during armed conflict.[41,42] These violations are: the recruitment and use of children by parties to armed conflict, their killing and maiming, rape and other forms of sexual violence, abductions of children, attacks on schools and hospitals, and denial of humanitarian access for children (**Box 2**). These violations were selected based on their suitability for monitoring and verification, their egregious nature, and the severity of their consequences on the lives of children. The use of the term "grave violations" refers to each individual child affected by recruitment and use, killing and maiming, sexual violence and abductions, and the number of incidents is used for attacks on schools and hospitals and the denial of humanitarian access.

The 6 grave violations against children are assessed by the United Nations on a yearly basis. In its 2020 report the United Nations verified more than 25,000 grave violations against children in 19 situations, more than one-half committed by nonstate actors, and one-third by government and international forces.[43] Overall, 24,422 violations were committed or continued to be committed in 2019 and 1241 were committed previously and verified in 2019. Because of the careful verification process that is followed, these numbers are almost certainly underestimates of the actual numbers.

Box 1
Countries where child soldiers are recruited

Central African Republic

Afghanistan

Democratic Republic of the Congo

Iraq

Myanmar

Nigeria

Somalia

South Sudan

Syrian Arab Republic

Yemen

Adapted from https://theirworld.org/news/10-countries-where-child-soldiers-are-still-recruited-in-armed-conflicts.

> **Box 2**
> **The 6 grave violations against children during armed conflict**
>
> 1. Recruitment and use of children
>
> 2. Killing or maiming of children
>
> 3. Sexual violence against children
>
> 4. Attacks against schools or hospitals
>
> 5. Abduction of children
>
> 6. Denial of humanitarian access

Recruitment and Use of Children as Soldiers

It is very difficult to know how many children are recruited and used as soldiers, but the annual report of the secretary general on children and armed conflict is 1 source of information. In its 2020 report, the United Nations verified that 7747 children, some as young as 6 years old, had been recruited and used as soldiers. Among those, 90% were used by nonstate actors.[43]

Killing and Maiming of Children

In its 2020 report, the United Nations verified that 4019 children were killed and 6154 children were maimed.[43] The deaths and injuries occurred because of crossfire, small arms and light weapons, ground engagement between parties, the use of explosive weapons in populated areas, and the excessive use of force by state actors. Afghanistan remained the deadliest conflict for children, with a 67% increase in suicide and complex attacks affecting children. In Myanmar, there was a 3-fold increase in child casualties; 25% were caused by explosive remnants of war, improvised explosive devices and antipersonnel mines. The highest prevalence of such casualties was in Iraq and the Philippines.

Rape and Other Forms of Sexual Violence

In 2019, the United Nations reported 735 verified cases of rape and other forms of sexual violence against children.[43] This number is considered to be vastly under-reported. Cases were prevalent in the Democratic Republic of the Congo, Somalia, the Central African Republic, the Sudan, and South Sudan. Cases attributed to state actors nearly doubled, reinforcing the fear of retaliations and of stigma for children and families willing to report sexual violence.

Abduction

In 2019, The United Nations verified the abduction of 1683 children, with more than 95% of cases perpetrated by nonstate actors, mainly in Somalia, the Democratic Republic of the Congo, and Nigeria.[43] Children were abducted for recruitment and use as soldiers, as well as sexual violence or ransom.

Attacks on Schools and Hospitals

In 2019, the United Nations verified 494 attacks on schools and 433 attacks on hospitals.[43] The highest numbers were verified in the Syrian Arab Republic, the Occupied Palestinian Territory, Afghanistan, and Somalia. Globally, there were 503 attacks on schools and hospitals committed by state actors; this number was nearly double the number in 2018. In many places in Gaza and Israel, schools were used for military purposes. When classes were not canceled indefinitely, classes were suspended for weeks or longer.

Denial of Humanitarian Access

In 2019, the United Nations verified some 4400 incidents of the denial of humanitarian access to children. Overwhelmingly, nonstate actors were responsible for such incidents, especially in Yemen, Mali, the Central African Republic, and the Syrian Arab Republic.[43]

GLOBAL PREVENTION EFFORTS

A total of 13,200 children were separated from nonstate actors and armed forces globally in 2019.[43] Comprehensive efforts have focused on successfully reintegrating them into society. The Global Coalition for the Reintegration of Former Child Soldiers is an alliance of Member States, United Nations entities, the World Bank, nongovernment organizations and academia launched in 2018 to advance global efforts to address reintegration of former child soldiers, and prompt action to increase children's access to sustainable, long-term support.[44]

During 2020, the twentieth anniversary of the Convention on the Rights of the Child—Children in Conflict, the United Nations took a number of initiatives with regard to consideration of children when negotiating peace agreements. This effort included publishing a set of guiding principles[45] to assist mediators in their consideration of child protection issues:

1. All children are equally entitled to all of the rights enshrined in the Convention on the Rights of the Child, at all times, in accordance with its article 2. No child should be discriminated against on the basis of the child's, or her or his parent's or legal guardian's gender, age, ethnicity, race, religion, physical abilities, or any other status.
2. In accordance with article 3 of the Convention, it is important to consider the best interests of children during peace negotiations in all decisions that will—directly or indirectly—affect them.
3. All actions undertaken and decisions made for the protection of children should respect the principle of "do no harm." Efforts should be made to minimize possible negative effects and maximize benefits for children, to ensure that their needs are met, and that, in accordance with their age and maturity, their views are heard, in a manner consistent with article 12 of the Convention. The inclusion of the viewpoints of children may be achieved by different means, including through community-based initiatives led by civil society or other stakeholders involved in the peace process.
4. Consistency should be ensured with the content and nature of the Convention on the Rights of the Child, the Optional Protocol to the Convention on the Rights of the Child on the involvement of children in armed conflict, Security Council resolutions on children and armed conflict, and relevant resolutions for the specific country concerned as applicable during the mediation effort, while recalling that the United Nations does not support amnesty for serious crimes under international law and that perpetrators of grave violations against children cannot be exempted from accountability.

It is time to end the recruitment and use of children under 18 years of age in armed conflicts. This condition has been called for in 2007 in the Paris Commitments,[46] which have been endorsed by 110 States.[47] There is much more to be done to stop making children into soldiers.

CLINICS CARE POINTS

- Complex consequences on both physical and mental health are reported among child soldiers.
- One-third to one-half of children affected by armed conflict may have clinically significant symptoms of PTSD.
- The recruitment and use of children in armed conflicts must stop.

DISCLOSURE

The author has nothing to disclose.

REFERENCES

1. War child. 2018. Why do children become child soldiers?. Available at: https://www.warchild.org.uk/whats-happening/features/why-do-children-become-child-soldiers-armed-groups. Accessed January 28, 2021..
2. Wessels MG. Child soldiers: from violence to prevention. Boston: Harvard University Press; 2006. p. 34.
3. Steinberg L. Cognitive and affective development in adolescence. Trends Cogn Sci 2005;9:69–74.
4. Junger E. Storm of steel. Translated by Michael Hofmann. New York: Penguin Books; 2016. p. 5.
5. Freedman R. The war to end all wars: World War I. Boston: Clarion Books; 2010. p. 42.
6. Abu-Hayyeh R, Singh G. Adverse health effects of recruiting child soldiers. BMJ Paediatr Open 2019;3(1):c000325.
7. Gee D, Goodman A. Young age at army enlistment is associated with greater war zone risks. Forces Watch 2013. Available at: https://www.forceswatch.net/sites/default/files/Young_age_at_army_enlistment_greater_risks%28FINAL%29.pdf.
8. Santa Barbara J. Impact of war on children and imperative to end war. Croat Med J 2006;47:891–4.
9. Jones M, Sundin J, Goodwin L, et al. What explains post-traumatic stress disorder (PTSD) in UK service personnel: deployment or something else? Psychol Med 2013;43:1703–12.
10. Ministry of Defence. UK armed forces suicide and open verdict deaths: 2016. 2017. Available at: https://www.gov.uk/government/statistics/uk-armed-forces-suicide-and-open-verdict-deaths-2016.
11. Hines LA, Jawahar K, Wessely S, et al. Self-harm in the UK military. Occup Med 2013;63:354–7. https://doi.org/10.1093/occmed/kqt065. Accessed January 28, 2021.
12. Buckman JE, Forbes HJ, Clayton T, et al. Early Service leavers: a study of the factors associated with premature separation from the UK Armed Forces and the mental health of those that leave early. Eur J Public Health 2013;23:410–5.
13. Gee D. The First Ambush? Effects of army training and employment. London, United Kingdom: Veterans for Peace; 2017. Available at: https://www.forceswatch.net/resources/the-first-ambush-effects-of-army-training-and-employment/.

14. Gee D. The Last Ambush? Aspects of mental health in the British armed forces. London: ForcesWatch; 2013. Available at: https://www.forceswatch.net/resources/the-last-ambush-aspects-of-mental-health-in-the-british-armed-forces/. Accessed January 28, 2021.
15. Hilton J. Lost Horizon. New York: William Morrow; 1933. p. 167.
16. Slone M, Mann S. Effects of war, terrorism and armed conflict on young children: a systematic review. Child Psychiatry Hum Dev 2016;47(6):950–65.
17. Betancourt TS, Borisova II, de la Soudière M, et al. Sierra Leone's child soldiers: war exposures and mental health problems by gender. J Adolesc Health 2011; 49(1):21–8.
18. Medeiros E, Shrestha PN, Gaire H, et al. Life after armed group involvement in Nepal: a clinical ethnography of psychological well-being of former "child soldiers" over time. Transcult Psychiatry 2020;57(1):183–96.
19. Kizilhan JI, Noll-Hussong M. Post-traumatic stress disorder among former Islamic State child soldiers in northern Iraq. Br J Psychiatry 2018;213(1):425–9.
20. Williams R. The Psychosocial Consequences for Children and Young People who are Exposed to Terrorism, War, Conflict and Natural Disasters. Curr Opin Psychiatry 2006;19(4):337–49.
21. Fisher J, Cabral de Mello M, Izutsu T, et al. Mental health and psychosocial consequences of armed conflict and natural disasters. Int J Soc Psychiatry 57, Suppl. 1:57–78.
22. Cieslak TJ, Henretig FM. Bioterrorism. Pediatr Ann 2003;32(3):154–65.
23. American Academy of Pediatrics Council on Environmental Health. Chapter 3: Children's unique vulnerabilities to environmental hazards. In: Etzel RA, editor. Pediatric environmental health. 4th Edition. Itasca (IL): American Academy of Pediatrics; 2019. p. 17–31.
24. Chung S, Baum CR, Nyquist A-C. AAP Disaster Preparedness Advisory Council, Council on Environmental Health, Committee on Infectious Diseases. Chemical-Biological Terrorism and Its Impact on Children. Pediatrics 2020;145(2): e20193750.
25. Rotenberg JS, Newmark J. Nerve agent attacks on children: diagnosis and management. Pediatrics 2003;112(3 Pt 1):648–58.
26. Nakajima T, Ohta S, Morita H, et al. Epidemiological study of sarin poisoning in Matsumoto City, Japan. J Epidemiol 1998;8(1):33–41 [Erratum appears in J Epidemiol 1998;8(2):129].
27. Khan K, Wozniak SE, Coleman J, et al. Wartime toxin exposure: recognising the silent killer. BMJ Case Rep 2016;2016. https://doi.org/10.1136/bcr-2016-217438.
28. Zwijnenburg W, Hochhauser D, Dewachi O, et al. Solving the jigsaw of conflict-related environmental damage: utilizing open-source analysis to improve research into environmental health risks. J Public Health (Oxf) 2020;42(3): e352–60.
29. Levy BS, Sidel VW. War, Terrorism, and Children's Health. In: Landrigan PJ, Etzel RA, editors. Chapter 58 in: Textbook of children's environmental health. New York: Oxford University Press; 2014. p. 537–45.
30. Vänskä M, Diab SY, Perko K, et al. Toxic environment of war: maternal prenatal heavy metal load predicts infant emotional development. Infant Behav Dev 2019;55:1–9.
31. United Nations Children's Fund (UNICEF). Healthy environments for healthy children: global programme framework. New York: UNICEF; 2021. p. 28. Available at: https://www.unicef.org/media/91216/file/Healthy-Environments-for-Healthy-Children-Global-Programme-Framework-2021.pdf. Accessed January 28, 2021.

32. Extensive data collection by the Armed Conflict Location & Event Data Project (ACLED). Available at: http://www.acleddata.com/dashboard/#dashboard. Accessed January 28, 2021.
33. Armstrong M. The World at War in 2020 [Digital image]. Retrieved January 28, 2021, from https://www.statista.com/chart/21652/countries-with-armed-clashes-reported/.
34. Machel G. The Impact of Armed Conflict on Children attached to: UN Note of the Secretary General, A/51/306. 1996. para. 317. Available at: https://www.un.org/ga/search/view_doc.asp?symbol=A/51/306. Accessed January 28, 2021.
35. Machel G. The impact of war on children. London: UNICEF; 2001.
36. Bhutta ZA, Yousafzai AK, Zipursky A. Pediatrics, war, and children. Curr Probl Pediatr Adolesc Health Care 2010;40:20–35.
37. Kadir A, Shenoda S, Goldhagen J, Pitterman S, Section on International Child Health. The effects of armed conflict on children. Pediatrics 2018;142(6): e20182586.
38. Song SJ, de Jong J. Child soldiers: children associated with fighting forces. Child Adolesc Psychiatr Clin N Am 2015;24(4):765–75.
39. Rieder M, Choonara I. Armed conflict and child health. Arch Dis Child 2012;97(1): 59–62.
40. Ten countries where child soldiers are still recruited in armed conflicts. 2017. Available at: https://reliefweb.int/report/central-african-republic/10-countries-where-child-soldiers-are-still-recruited-armed.
41. Office of the Special Representative of the Secretary-General for Children and Armed Conflict. The Six Grave Violations Against Children During Armed Conflict: The Legal Foundation October 2009 (Updated November 2013). Available at: https://childrenandarmedconflict.un.org/publications/WorkingPaper-1_SixGraveViolationsLegalFoundation.pdf. Accessed January 28, 2021.
42. UNICEF, United Nations Office of the Special Representative of the Secretary-General for Children and Armed Conflict. Machel study 10-year strategic review: children and conflict in a changing world. 2009. Available at: https://www.unicef.org/publications/%20index_49985.html. Accessed November 13, 2020.
43. United Nations Secretary General. Children and armed conflict. Report of the Secretary-General. 2020. (A/74/845–S/2020/525). Available at: https://childrenandarmedconflict.un.org/publications/MachelStudy-10YearStrategicReview_en.pdf. Accessed January 28, 2021.
44. Global Coalition for the Reintegration of Former Child Soldiers. Improving Support to Child Reintegration Summary of findings from three reports. 2020. Available at: https://childrenandarmedconflict.un.org/wp-content/uploads/2020/03/GCR-Reintegration-Summary-paper-February-2020.pdf. Accessed January 28, 2021.
45. United Nations Office of the Special Representative of the Secretary-General for Children and Armed Conflict. Practical guidance for mediators to protect children in situations of armed conflict. 2020. Available at: https://childrenandarmedconflict.un.org/wp-content/uploads/2020/07/Practical-guidance-for-mediators-to-protect-children-in-situations-of-armed-conflict.pdf. Accessed January 28, 2021.
46. The Paris Commitments to protect children from unlawful recruitment or use by armed forces or armed groups. 2007. Available at: https://childrenandarmedconflict.un.org/publications/ParisCommitments_EN.pdf. Accessed January 28, 2021.
47. Permanent Delegation of France. Available at: https://onu.delegfrance.org/Children-and-armed-conflicts-10458. Accessed January 28, 2021.

Addressing Violence Against Children Through Anti-racism Action

Camara Phyllis Jones, MD, MPH, PhD[a,b,c,*]

KEYWORDS

- Racism • Anti-racism • Racism denial

KEY POINTS

- Racism is a system of structuring opportunity and assigning value based on the social interpretation of how one looks (which is what we call "race").
- Racism unfairly disadvantages some individuals and communities, unfairly advantages other individuals and communities, and saps the strength of the whole society through the waste of human resources.
- There are 7 barriers to achieving health equity that are deeply embedded in US culture. These serve as values targets for anti-racism action.
- Four of these undergird this nation's staunch racism denial: our narrow focus on the individual, a-historical stance, myth of meritocracy, and White supremacist ideology.
- Three others stymy efforts to assure the conditions for optimal health for all people: Our limited future orientation, myth of a zero-sum game, and myth of American exceptionalism.

Editor's comment: This article is written from a deeply personal perspective that is then elevated to the values to be targeted in action steps guiding policy and practice. In framing the discussion of ending the violence against children, 2 principles must guide our actions: the rights of children and our determination to eliminate racism.

—Danielle Laraque-Arena, MD, FAAP.

If we are truly concerned about the future of humanity and the survival of our species on this planet, we must dismiss any distinctions between "my" children and "your" children

[a] Department of Behavioral Sciences and Health Education, Rollins School of Public Health, Emory University, Atlanta, GA, USA; [b] Department of Epidemiology, Rollins School of Public Health, Emory University, Atlanta, GA, USA; [c] Department of Community Health and Preventive Medicine and Satcher Health Leadership Institute, Morehouse School of Medicine, Atlanta, GA, USA
* 826 Oakdale Road NE, Atlanta, GA 30307.
E-mail address: cpjones@msm.edu
Twitter: @CamaraJones (C.P.J.)

Pediatr Clin N Am 68 (2021) 449–453
https://doi.org/10.1016/j.pcl.2021.01.002
0031-3955/21/© 2021 Elsevier Inc. All rights reserved.

to recognize that ALL children are "our" children.[1,2] Recognizing that violence against children includes not only physical violence and emotional violence but also the violence of deprivation and the violence of constrained dreams, we must recognize that racism is a system of power that perpetrates and perpetuates violence against children.

Racism is a system of structuring opportunity and assigning value based on the social interpretation of how one looks (which is what we call "race"), that unfairly disadvantages some individuals and communities, unfairly advantages other individuals and communities, and saps the strength of the whole society through the waste of human resources.[3,4]

There are many pearls in that one-sentence definition: First, that racism is a system, not an individual character flaw, not a personal moral failing, not even a psychiatric illness, but a system of power; second, that so-called "race", the substrate on which racism operates, is not in our genes but is the social interpretation of how one looks in a "race"-conscious society; third, that racism has 3 impacts, unfairly disadvantaging some while unfairly advantaging other individuals and communities, but also sapping the strength of the whole society through the waste of human resources; and finally, that racism operates in 2 ways, both by structuring opportunity and by assigning value.

We recognize that we must address BOTH the differential opportunity structures and the differential value assignment in order to dismantle racism.

We already know many of the *structural targets* for anti-racism action in the context of the United States[5,6]: residential segregation and disinvestment by "race"; funding of public schools based on local property taxes with resultant educational and occupational segregation by "race"; overpolicing of communities of color, disproportionate police violence against communities of color, and lack of accountability of police officers or departments; disproportionate incarceration of black and brown men and women; consignment of communities of color to serve as environmental "sacrifice zones"; lack of reparations to descendants of Africans enslaved in the United States. Anti-racism activists are rightfully targeting their efforts toward redressing these historical and contemporary structural factors and revealing inaction in the face of need.[7,8]

However, we may have so far neglected many possible *values targets* for anti-racism action.[9] I would like to present the following 7 candidates for our consideration:

- Limited future orientation
- Narrow focus on the individual
- A-historical stance
- Myth of meritocracy
- Myth of a zero-sum game
- Myth of American exceptionalism
- White supremacist ideology

Four of these directly contribute to the staunch racism denial so prevalent in the United States (and other nations): our narrow focus on the individual, a-historical stance, myth of meritocracy, and White supremacist ideology. Three others stymy efforts to assure the conditions for optimal health for all people: our limited future orientation, myth of a zero-sum game, and myth of American exceptionalism. All 7 inhibit our ability to create a society in which all children can know and have the opportunity to develop to their full potentials. This represents a societal-level form of violence against children.

LIMITED FUTURE ORIENTATION

The connection between racism, these 7 values targets for anti-racism action, and the many forms of violence against children is most blatantly manifest in our *limited future orientation.* There are 2 parts of the future that each of us can touch today: the first, the children and the second, the planet. In the United States, we exhibit a flagrant disregard for the children. We do not have the "seven generations hence" perspective that many American Indian nations have when they consider the impacts of their decisions. Nor do we have a "How are the children?" focus like many East African peoples do when they greet one another with the question, "How are the children?" and hope to get the response, "All the children are well." Indeed, we rarely inquire about the well-being of our nation's children, and when we do, we certainly do not get the answer that "All the children are well." The impact of our lack of future orientation with regard to the children is compounded by our usurious relationship with the planet.

This lack of future orientation is critical to overturn. Both the children themselves and the future that they represent must be nurtured, respected, and prioritized in national and local policies. The violence toward children in the United States and worldwide reveals a fundamental flaw in our societal structures and values. The lack of caring for the planet that our children will inherit displays a fundamental gap in our societal consciousness and collective responsibility to care for one another. Our limited future orientation blinds us to the prudence of investing in the safety, protection, and nurturing of all the children and the planet as an investment in the survival of the species.

NARROW FOCUS ON THE INDIVIDUAL

It follows that the limited future orientation may be tied to a *narrow focus on the individual*, a decidedly selfish view of the world. In the United States and in some places around the world, we are so narrowly focused on the individual that it makes systems and structures invisible or seemingly irrelevant. Our sense of self-interest is very narrowly defined, often including only our immediate households and not even extending to aunts, uncles, and cousins, much less to neighbors or to strangers across town. Many of us do not have a sense of interdependence, that "There but for the grace of God go I" or "We're all in this together." This narrow focus on the individual also constrains our effectiveness in trying to change things, because we ask ourselves, "What can I do?" as rugged individuals, instead of understanding the power of collective action and asking, "What can WE do?" together.

A-HISTORICAL STANCE

In the United States and globally, we are ahistorical, acting as if the present were disconnected from the past and as if the current distribution of advantage and disadvantage were just a happenstance. Being a-historical also constrains our understanding of how to make change happen. If things were a certain way when we were born, we assume that they have always been that way and will always be that way. If we do not fully understand how things came to be the way they are or learn from the history of past movements for change, our current view of what is possible and how to build a better future will be limited.

MYTH OF MERITOCRACY

The national admonishment to "Pull yourself up by your bootstraps," the celebration of the Horatio Alger story, the insistence (most notably in the United States) that this is the land of equal opportunity: these are all vigorous endorsements of the myth of meritocracy, that "If you work hard, you will make it." I give you that most people who have made it in this country have worked hard. (Mind you, not all people who have made it have worked hard, and we currently have prominent examples of some exceptions.) However, even as we acknowledge that most people who have made it have worked hard, we must also recognize that there are many, many other people who are working just as hard, or harder, who will never make it because of an uneven playing field. That uneven playing field has been structured and is being maintained by racism, sexism, heterosexism, capitalism, and other systems of structured inequity.

To the extent that we deny racism, we are endorsing the myth of meritocracy and blaming folks who do not make it, labeling them as lazy or stupid. There are many ways to deny racism. One way is to say, "Racism does not exist." Another way is to never say the word "racism." Because even if we are talking about "disparities" or "disproportionalities" or "diversity, equity, and inclusion" or "implicit or unconscious bias" or "cultural competence" or "structural competence" or even "race," if we never say the word "racism" in our national context of widespread racism denial, we are complicit with that denial.

MYTH OF A ZERO-SUM GAME

The zero-sum game is the myth that "If you gain, I lose," which fosters competition over cooperation, masks the costs of inequity (the reality that racism is sapping the strength of the whole society through the waste of human resources), and hinders efforts to grow the pie. It is as if I do not want you to come to my dinner table because I think that you will just come and eat up all of the food, without recognizing that you are bringing all kinds of cakes and pies and roasts and fruits and salads with you. It comes from 2 deeply held beliefs, that you have nothing of value to offer and that I have everything that I need at my table. Neither of those beliefs is ever true. Each of us has something to teach, and each of us has something to learn.

MYTH OF AMERICAN EXCEPTIONALISM

American exceptionalism is the myth that the United States is so special, so different, so unique, so blessed by God that the rules for others may not apply to us. (This sentiment is likely expressed similarly in other countries.) Endorsement of this myth gives us a false sense of entitlement and makes us disinterested in learning from the experiences of other nations. Although this attitude may not be unique to the United States, it is important that we drop our false pride and learn from how other countries are more successfully handling the current COVID-19 pandemic. Hundreds of thousands of lives would have already been saved. Our families would not be so devastated; our communities would not be in such crisis, and we would still have access to the lost genius and leadership that could have helped the nation and the world navigate this global crisis.

WHITE SUPREMACIST IDEOLOGY

White supremacist ideology is the false belief that there exists a hierarchy of human valuation by "race" and that puts "White" people at the top of this fictional hierarchy as the ideal and the norm. This ideology has given people who are living as "white" a sense of entitlement, resulted in the dehumanization of people of color, and led to the fear by some at the "browning of America" that underlies much of our political divide today.

Where do we go from here?

Approaches to addressing these 7 values targets will involve all of us. We need to augment our curricula at all levels of education to name racism and other systems of structured inequity and prevent another generation from being lulled into the somnolence of racism denial. We need to teach our full histories. We need to change the media practices that make some of us at times invisible and at other times hypervisible. Perhaps our religious institutions will need to get involved. We will need to burst through our bubbles of experience to realize that folks across town are just as kind, funny, generous, hard-working, and smart as we are, but are living in very different circumstances. We need to become interested in the stories of others, believe the stories of others, and then join in the stories of others. We must be especially mindful of our children, our responsibility vis-à-vis their welfare, and that violence of every kind, physical, emotional, or economic, limits their future and is unjust.

This article and this special issue are an invitation to all of us who love children to join in and become actively anti-racism. Racism structures opportunities that differentially allow or constrain children from developing to their full potentials. Racism assigns value that differentially celebrates or dehumanizes children and frame their understandings of their full potentials. But perhaps most importantly, racism saps the strength of the whole society through the waste of human resources. Our children are our human resource. All our children. We must protect their precious genius and full humanity with all that we have, because they are all that we have.

CLINICS CARE POINTS

- Anti-racism action is a legitimate and necessary role for health care providers.
- A National Campaign Against Racism has the following 3 tasks:
  - Name racism
  - Ask "How is racism operating here?"
  - Organize and strategize to act

DISCLOSURE

The author has nothing to disclose.

REFERENCES

1. Jones CP, Jones CY, Perry GS, et al. Addressing the social determinants of children's health: a cliff analogy. J Health Care Poor Underserved 2009;20(4 Suppl):1–12.
2. Jones CP. Pondering the meaning of life: 'And how are the children?'. Nations Health 2016;46:3.
3. Jones CP. Confronting institutionalized racism. Phylon 2003;50(1–2):7–22.
4. Jones CP, Truman BI, Elam-Evans LD, et al. Using "socially-assigned race" to probe white advantages in health status. Ethn Dis 2008;18(4):496–504.
5. Jones CP. Levels of racism: a theoretic framework and a gardener's tale. Am J Public Health 2000;90(8):1212–5.
6. Jones CP. "Race", racism, and the practice of epidemiology. Am J Epidemiol 2001; 154(4):299–304.
7. Jones CP. Systems of power, axes of inequity: parallels, intersections, braiding the strands. Med Care 2014;52(10 Suppl 3):S71–5.
8. Jones CP. Toward the science and practice of anti-racism: launching a national campaign against racism. Ethn Dis 2018;28(Suppl 1):231–4.
9. Jones CP. Seeing the water: seven values targets for anti-racism action. Harv Prim Care Blog 2020. Available at: http://info.primarycare.hms.harvard.edu/blog/seven-values-targets-anti-racism-action. Accessed August 25, 2020.

Domestic Violence and Its Effects on Women, Children, and Families

Ingrid Walker-Descartes, MD, MPH, MBA[a],*, Madeline Mineo, DO[a],
Luisa Vaca Condado, BA[a], Nina Agrawal, MD[b]

KEYWORDS

- Domestic violence • Intimate partner violence • Child abuse
- Pandemic preparedness

KEY POINTS

- There are significant mental and physical health consequences for all members in a household with an established culture of violence.
- Any level of exposure to violence in any form is associated with considerable impairment in children similar to other forms of child abuse and maltreatment.
- Families with an established culture of violence experience heightened vulnerabilities during pandemics and natural disasters; therefore, resources tailored to the needs of these families must be publicized during these times of intense stress.

INTRODUCTION

Domestic violence (DV) and intimate partner violence (IPV), despite an overlap in their dynamics and impact, are different. By definition, DV takes place within a household and can involve a parent and child, siblings, or even roommates.[1] IPV occurs between romantic partners who may or may not be living together. It is "physical, sexual or psychological harm by a current or former partner or spouse which includes any incident of violent or threatening behavior or abuse between adults in heterosexual or same-sex relationships."[2] Neither IPV or DV is limited to physical aggression (ie, hitting, kicking, and beating), but IPV also encompasses emotional abuse (ie, intimidation or controlling actions with the desired endpoint of isolation from family and friends or financial control).[1] Both forms of violence also fall within a continuum of violence occurring in a household.

Exposure to DV/ IPV is a form of child maltreatment. In light of the overlap and despite the differences between these terms, they will be used interchangeably

[a] Department of Pediatrics, Maimonides Children's Hospital of Brooklyn, 4802 Tenth Avenue, Brooklyn, NY 11219, USA; [b] City University of New York (CUNY) - Graduate School of Public Health and Health Policy, 235 West 102nd Street, New York, NY 10025, USA
* Corresponding author.
E-mail address: lwalker-descartes@maimonidesmed.org

Pediatr Clin N Am 68 (2021) 455–464
https://doi.org/10.1016/j.pcl.2020.12.011
0031-3955/21/© 2021 Elsevier Inc. All rights reserved.

throughout this content with the consideration that children's exposure, whether witnessed or not, results in a significant amount of impairment. A child's awareness that a caregiver is being harmed or is at risk of harm is sufficient to induce harmful sequelae.[3,4] The term, exposure to IPV or DV, is used as the most inclusive term with no distinction between children who have witnessed versus those that have suffered direct physical injury from DV or IPV.

According to the 2011 National Intimate Partner and Sexual Violence Survey, 71.4% of women and 58.2% of men who were victims of IPV had their first incident before the age of 25, with 23.2% of women and 14.1% of men having occurred before the age of 18.[5] Women are at least 3 times more likely than men to experience injury from partner violence, although, in the United States, 13.8% of men also have experienced severe IPV at some point.[6] In 2010, IPV contributed to 1295 deaths, accounting for 10% of all homicides for that year.[6] Prevalence data likely are a gross underestimate, because many cases of IPV go unreported.[6,7]

DISCUSSION
The Impact on Women

Female householder families, defined as a household where a girl who is older than 15 years old is the responsible party, remains on the rise since the 1940s. The US Census Bureau reported approximately 3410 families in the 1940s to approximately 15,043 families as of 2019.[8] In these cases, census records define that the occupied housing unit is rented or owned by a woman and the family consists of individuals where at least 1 individual is related to the householder by birth, marriage, or adoption.[8] Therefore, the impact of IPV/DV has far-reaching implications for the physical and mental health of not only the woman but also all members of the family. In worst-case scenarios, it determines the mechanism of death for its victims. Homicide often is the tragic endpoint of many battering relationships. In the United States, women are killed by intimate partners more often than by any other type of perpetrator, with approximately 1 out of 5 murder victims killed by an intimate partner.[9–13] IPV homicides accounts for approximately 40% to 50% of femicides—the intentional murder of women because they are women.[11,14–17] Additionally, a majority (67%–80%) of intimate partner homicides involve physical abuse of the woman by her male partner before the murder, no matter if the woman or her male partner is killed, while a crucial household factor contributing to the escalation of nonfatal spouse abuse to homicide is having a gun in the home.[12,13,18]

The Impact on Physical Health

DV threatens the physical health of its victims. Data from the National Electronic Injury Surveillance System–All Injury Program used to trend the fracture patterns of IPV patients in the United States reported 1.65 million emergency department visits over 9 years for injuries related to DV.[19] A majority of the victims were women (83.3%), with contusion/abrasions (43.4%), lacerations (16.9%), strain/sprains (15.6%), internal organ injuries (14.4%), and fractures (9.7%) among the major diagnoses. The most common fracture involved the face (48.3%), followed by the finger (9.9%), upper trunk (9.8%), and hand (6.4%).[19] Studies focused on increasing the physician's index of suspicion for DV revealed patterns of injury involving central injuries to the head, neck, chest/thorax, abdomen, and perineum were reported to be the most common among victims of DV, with the head the most common site (78%) for lethal DV gunshot wounds.[20] Despite anatomic and physiologic differences between adults and children, similar injuries seen in infants who experienced shaking as a result of their abuse may be observed in adult female victims presenting with retinal hemorrhages, subdural hematoma, and patterned bruising after an episode of DV.[21] Head injuries also predominate as the most common injury documented on ED visits preceding homicides related to DV—a trend that also holds for infant victims of abusive head trauma.[19,21–23]

The Impact on Mental Health

The psychological impact of IPV/DV can be insidious but no less debilitating than the physical sequelae. Early theories speculated that this type of violence was the product of mental illness; however, research continues to validate that mental illness is an unavoidable consequence rather than a contributor.[24] The mental health impact is experienced as part of the spectrum of abusive behaviors known as psychological violence and as the sequelae to the other forms of DV/IPV. Psychological violence includes 3 broad categories of manipulation, isolation, and intimidation. Specific behaviors include abandonment or ill treatment; threats; home-based isolation; intimidation of children's removal; separation from the support systems, such as family; public offenses or insults; verbal aggression; economic deprivations; and obsessive surveillance (ie, stalking).[25] Most research addressing the consequences of IPV has focused on acts of physical aggression, whereas less attention has been paid to the difficult to measure dimensions of psychological abuse.[25] Despite this challenge, the focus on mental health outcomes for victims must be weighted similarly. This is important especially because battered women frequently identify psychological abuse as inflicting greater distress compared with physical acts of violence.[25,26]

In a study to identify posttraumatic psychiatric morbidity associated with DV, a sample of 335 women were recruited to establish baseline data.[27] The outcome measures of lifetime psychiatric diagnoses showed that women who reported lifetime adult intimate abuse (n = 162) received significantly more diagnoses of generalized anxiety, dysthymia, depression, phobias, current harmful alcohol consumption, and psychoactive drug dependence than those who reported no abuse (n = 173).[27] Of the 191 women tested for lifetime posttraumatic stress disorder (PTSD), those who reported lifetime abuse (n = 115) received significantly more diagnoses than those who reported no abuse (n = 76), with measurement of the population-attributable risk finding that one-third of the psychiatric diagnoses were attributable to DV.[27] Although the mechanisms by which partner violence lead to diminished functioning have yet to be definitively established, evidence suggests that chronic posttraumatic and depressive symptoms may contribute substantially to the decline in a women's functioning.[28,29] Mechanic and collegues'[30] study highlighting the importance of examining multiple dimensions of intimate partner abuse and mental health outcomes revealed PTSD and depression tended to be highly comorbid, thereby further increasing the likelihood of debilitating outcomes. Recovery from these mental health sequelae of DV, specifically PTSD and depression, can be hampered further by the social determinants of health linked to poverty. Lack of material and social resources may exacerbate parenting stress and other stressors secondary to partner abuse or separation from an abusive relationship.[31–33] Repeat abuse over time also is more likely to occur among battered women with the fewest resources, whereas social support appeared a protective factor.[7,33–35]

Impact of Domestic Violence/Intimate Partner Violence on Children at Different Developmental Stages

Violence in the household increases a child's risk of maltreatment as a culture of violence is established within that household. Statistics are consistent in that approximately 26% to 73% of families reported to have child abuse present also are affected by IPV, whereas approximately 30% to 60% of families reported to have IPV present also are affected by child abuse.[36] Children's exposure to violence occur in a variety of ways: (1) witnessing violence, (2) hearing but not observing the violence, (3) observing the aftermath (seeing bruises on the mother, broken furniture, and so forth), (4) becoming aware of the violence (someone else tells them about it), and (5) living in a household in which violence occurs but not being aware of it.[37] No matter the exposure, children and adolescents are deeply impacted by these experiences because 30% to 60% of men who abuse their female partner also abuse their children.[38–42] Most children from violent families witness their fathers or other male authority figure assaulting their mothers. Some abusers may arrange for the child to be present to witness the violence as a visible statement of their authority.[43] This exposure may leave permanent sequelae that can greatly interfere with a child's physical and emotional development. Approximately half of all children exposed to DV have emotional and behavioral problems in the clinical range and are in need of behavioral health services with varied presentations across their age ranges.[44–46]

Infants, toddlers, and preschoolers
Young children depend on their caretakers to meet their needs for safety and security. Violence in the household undermines these needs, interfering with a child's normal development of trust and later exploratory behavior that leads to autonomy.[47] Because younger children do not have the verbal skills to express their feelings adequately, infants and toddlers who witness violence in their homes show excessive irritability, regressed behavior, sleep disturbances, emotional distress, and fear of being alone.[48] Older preschool children often present with psychosomatic problems, such as headaches, stomach aches, or being extremely fearful, with sleep disturbances, including insomnia, nightmares, sleepwalking, and enuresis.[49–51] Mothers of children in this age group report more behavioral problems than any other age group.[48] Children at this stage also are at increased risk for physical injuries sustained secondary to violence between adults. In a study where approximately 48% of the cohort were below 2 years old, the most common mechanism of injury was a direct hit, with a majority of injuries to the head (25%), face (19%), and eyes (18%).[48] Young children sustained more head and facial injuries than older children in this cohort because a common practice to block a forceful blow is to hold a child up as a shield.[48]

School-aged children
School-aged children are expected to explore, play freely, and show motivation to master their environment.[52] Children exposed to IPV/DV at this stage often show a greater frequency of internalizing symptoms (withdrawal and anxiety) as well as externalizing behavior problems (aggressiveness and delinquency) in comparison to children from nonviolent families.[46] Social competence and school performances often decline with an increase in sleep disturbances.[53] Preadolescent children may show a loss of interest in social activities, low self-esteem, withdrawal from or avoidance of peers, and disruptive behavior in the classroom. Older school-aged children exposed to violence seem to adopt a strategy of vigilance. These children appeared more responsive to aggressive information relative to nonaggressive cues and often attempted to intervene in fights, with a majority presenting disproportionately with extremity trauma.[49] In contrast, the younger children in this age group appear likely to narrow their information processing, discard aggressive information, and ignore or misinterpret social cues.[46,53]

Adolescents
Adolescence is a time of rapid physical, psychological, and social developmental changes. Along with the physical changes associated with puberty, adolescents are

expected to develop abstract thinking capacities, develop a clearer sense of their identities (ie, personal and sexual), and leverage their independence (ie, emotional, personal, and possibly financial).[54] All interactions with adolescents must be seen against this dynamic background of development where the adolescent is viewed within a system. Their position in the system is determined by their relationships with their parents, peers, and community. As adolescents begin to redefine themselves, they begin to define other people in relation to themselves.[54] When trauma is introduced into this system, adolescents are equipped with greater cognitive skills than their younger counterparts. This requires them to reconsider their roles and responsibilities to decide that certain events are not acceptable, should be stopped from happening, or should be reported to others who can help.[46,54] As a result, the adolescent becomes the victim of the assault when they intervene to defend or protect the victim. With continued exposure, adolescents often begin demonstrating high levels of aggression and acting out—a major risk factor for academic failure, school truancy, delinquency, and possible substance abuse.[53–55]

Screening

According to the National Academy of Medicine, "asking about interpersonal and DV experiences could identify abuse not otherwise detected, help prevent future abuse, lessen disability, and improve future functioning and success in life."[56] Some physicians rarely screen whereas others screen only when there are physical injuries.[57] In reality, many victims may not disclose abuse unless directly questioned under safe and respectful conditions.[58] American Academy of Pediatrics clinical practice guidelines recommend universal screening because pediatricians are in a unique position to recognize abused women in pediatric settings.[59,60] The use of direct or indirect questions is recommended. The approach depends on the type of clinical setting, provider style, relationship to the parent, perception and preference of the family, and potentially age of child in the room.[61,62] Utilizing an indirect approach a provider may open with, "I have begun to ask all of the caregivers in my practice about their family life as it affects their health and safety, and that of their children. May I ask you a few questions?"[62] Or a more direct approach may be, "Has your child witnessed a violent or frightening event in your home?"[62] Regardless of approach, it is optimal to ask about DV/IPV without the child in the room. Should a child be exposed to violence, a child safety assessment should be conducted. This consists of examining the child for physical abuse or neglect and determining if the child has been directly threatened and if the abused partner has a plan to keep the child safe. If there are indications that a child has been harmed or is in danger, a report to the state's central for child maltreatment is indicated. If this report is made, the caregiver always should be told.[62]

Considerations

Pandemics unmask areas of existing need for vulnerable populations. Women and children impacted by violence along the DV/IPV spectrum are no different. Prioritizing these needs, the Center for Global Development put forth the "Pandemics and Violence against Women and Children" (VAW/C) statement in April 2020, outlining strategies to maximize support to these families.[63] Pushing the integration of VAW/C programming into longer-term pandemic preparedness, incorporating a gender and age lens and ensuring women and children are included in preparedness processes, the guidelines highlight the following:

1. Bolster violence-related first-response systems: increasing staff or temporary operations for existing violence prevention and response hotlines and outreach

centers—increasing communication and awareness of services through routine news and advocacy for pandemic-specific contingencies around family conflict, divorce, and violence.[63]

2. Ensure VAW/C is integrated into health systems response: health care providers should be trained in identifying women at risk of violence present in all testing/screening locations, assessing the safety of recommendations for self-quarantine or shelter at home.[63]

3. Expand and reinforce social safety nets: proposals for rapid expansion of pro-poor social safety nets, including paid sick leave, unemployment insurance, direct cash or food voucher payments, and/or tax relief, are options.[63]

4. Expand shelter and temporary housing: temporary shelter and transitional housing for survivors of violence are likely to be reduced during pandemics. Although the sick, homeless, incarcerated, and other vulnerable populations also may be at high risk, ensuring pandemic-safe surge housing for high-risk women and children should remain a priority.[63]

Leveraging existing online and virtual platforms also can play a significant role during pandemics. Notable examples include myPlan from the United States, isafe in New Zealand, iCAN in Canada, and SAFE in the Netherlands.[64–67] In settings without options for online platforms, options for text-based networks such as WhatsApp can be maximized, building on existing women's groups and collectives.[67] These mechanisms may help women and children feel connected and supported, ameliorating the sense of isolation as they maintain their social networks.

SUMMARY

Children should be raised in a safe environment that protects from the emotional, cognitive, behavioral, and somatic problems associated with witnessing violence. Health care professionals can screen, identify, and manage this pathology in affected families while educating communities to the pernicious effects of exposure to violence along the DV/IPV continuum. These efforts will prove to address the larger public health issue—the establishment of a culture of violence in vulnerable households.

CLINICS CARE POINTS

- DV and IPV contribute equally to the establishment of a culture of violence in vulnerable households.

- Providers can screen for the existence of this culture of violence by adapting current DV/IPV screening tools.

- Women and children remain particularly vulnerable when there is the presence of a gun in the household—a key contributor to the escalation of DV/IPV to homicide.

- Pandemic preparedness plans must include surge planning for women and children affected by DV/IPV including an assessment of the safety of shelter in place orders for this vulnerable population.

DISCLOSURE

The authors have nothing to disclose.

REFERENCES

1. Moorer O. Intimate partner violence vs. domestic violence. 2019. Available at: https://ywcaspokane.org/what-is-intimate-partner-domestic-violence/. Accessed August 5, 2020.
2. Centers for Disease Control and Prevention. Intimate partner violence 2018. Available at: https://www.cdc.gov/violenceprevention/intimatepartnerviolence/index.html. Accessed August 5, 2020.
3. Wathen CN, Macmillan HL. Children's exposure to intimate partner violence: impacts and interventions. Paediatr Child Health 2013;18(8):419–22.
4. McTavish JR, MacGregor JCD, Wathen CN, et al. Children's exposure to intimate partner violence: an overview. Int Rev Psychiatry 2016;28(5):504–18.
5. Breiding MJ, Smith SG, Basile KC, et al. Prevalence and characteristics of sexual violence, stalking, and intimate partner violence victimization—national intimate sexual violence survey, United States, 2011. MMWR 2014;63(SS08):1–18. Available at: https://www.cdc.gov/mmwr/pdf/ss/ss6308.pdf. Accessed April 27, 2020.
6. Spivak HR, Jenkins EL, Van Audenhove K, et al. CDC grand rounds: a public health approach to prevention of intimate partner violence. MMWR 2014;63(2): 38–41. Available at: https://www.cdc.gov/mmwr/pdf/wk/mm6302.pdf. Accessed April 27, 2020.
7. Zolotor AJ, Denham AC, Weil A. Intimate partner violence. Obstet Gynecol Clin North Am 2009;36(4):847–60.
8. U.S. Census Bureau. Family households with female householder. In: FRED, Federal Reserve Bank of St. Louis. Available at: https://fred.stlouisfed.org/series/OFHHFH. Accessed June 29, 2020.
9. Cooper A, Smith E. Homicide trends in the United States, 1980-2008. Bureau of Justice 2011. Available at: https://www.bjs.gov/content/pub/pdf/htus8008.pdf. Accessed June 29, 2020.
10. Campbell JC, Webster D, Koziol-Mclain J, et al. Risk factors for femicide in abusive relationships: results from a multisite case control study. Am J Public Health 2003;93(7):1089–97.
11. Bailey JE, Kellermann AL, Somes GW, et al. Risk factors for violent death of women in the home. Arch Intern Med 1997;157:777–82.
12. Greenfield LA, Rand MR, Craven D, et al. Violence by Intimates: analysis of data on crimes by current or former spouses, boyfriends, and girlfriends. Washington, DC: US Department of Justice; 1998.
13. Langford L, Isaac NE, Kabat S. Homicides related to intimate partner violence in Massachusetts: Examining Case Ascertainment and Validity of the SHR. Homicide Stud 1998;2:353–77.
14. Frye V, Hosein V, Waltermaurer, et al. Femicide in New York City: 1990–1999. Homicide Stud 2005;9(3):204–28.
15. National Institute of Justice. A study of homicide in eight US Cities: an NIJ Intramural research Project. Washington, DC: US Dept of Justice; 1997.
16. McFarlane J, Campbell JC, Wilt S, et al. Stalking and intimate partner femicide. Homicide Stud 1999;3(4):300–16.
17. Violence Policy Center. When men murder women: an analysis of 2017 homicide data. 2019. Available at: https://vpc.org/studies/wmmw2019.pdf. Accessed August 5, 2020.
18. Loder RT, Momper L. Demographics and fracture patterns of patients presenting to US emergency departments for intimate partner violence. J Am Acad Orthop Surg Glob Res Rev 2020;4(2). e20.00009.

19. Wadman MC, Muelleman RL. Domestic violence homicides: ED use before victimization. Am J Emerg Med 1999;17(7):689–91.

20. Carrigan TD, Walker W, Barnes S. Domestic violence: the shaken adult syndrome. J Accid Emerg Med 2000;17(2):138–9.

21. Frasier LD, Kelly P, Al-Eissa M, et al. International issues in abusive head trauma. Pediatr Radiol 2014;44(Suppl 4):S647–53.

22. Roberts GL, Lawrence JM, Williams GM. The impact of domestic violence on women's mental health. Aust N Z J Public Health 1998;22(7):769–801.

23. Caponnetto P, Maglia M, Pistritto L, et al. Family violence and its psychological management at the emergency department: a review. Health Psychol Res 2019;7(2):8558.

24. Arias I. Women's responses to physical and psychological abuse. In: Arriaga XB, Oskamp S, editors. Violence in intimate relationships. Thousand Oaks (CA): Sage; 1999. p. 139–61.

25. Follingstad DR, Rutledge LL, Berg BJ, et al. The role of emotional abuse in physically abusive relationships. J Fam Viol 1990;5:107–20.

26. Vitanza S, Vogel LCM, Marshall LL. Distress and symptoms of posttraumatic stress disorder in abused women. Violence Vict 1995;10:23–34.

27. Mechanic MB. Beyond PTSD: mental health consequences of violence against women: a response to Briere and Jordan. J Interpers Violence 2004;19(11): 1283–9.

28. Sutherland C, Bybee D, Sullivan C. The long-term effects of battering on women's health. Women Health 1998;4:41–70.

29. Sutherland C, Bybee D, Sullivan C. Beyond bruises and broken bones: the joint effects of stress and injuries on battered women's health. Am J Community Psychol 2002;30(5):609–36.

30. Mechanic MB, Weaver TL, Resick PA. Mental health consequences of intimate partner abuse: a multidimensional assessment of four different forms of abuse. Violence Against Women 2008;14(6):634–54.

31. Anderson DK, Saunders DG, Mieko Y, et al. Long-term trends in depression among women separated from abusive partners. Violence Against Women 2003;9(7):807–38.

32. Ham-Rowbottom KA, Gordon EE, Jarvis KL, et al. Life constraints and psychological well-being of domestic violence shelter graduates. J Fam Viol 2005;20: 109–21.

33. Goodman L, Dutton MA, Vankos N, et al. Women's resources and use of strategies as risk and protective factors for reabuse over time. Violence Against Women 2005;11(3):311–36.

34. Sullivan CM, Basta J, Tan C, et al. After the crisis: a needs assessment of women leaving a domestic violence shelter. Violence Vict 1992;7(3):267–75.

35. Fanslow JL, Norton RN, Spinola CG. Indicators of assault-related injuries among women presenting to the emergency department. Ann Emerg Med 1998;32(3 Pt 1):341–8.

36. Flannery D, Huff CR. Youth violence: prevention, intervention, and social policy. Washington, DC: American Psychiatric Press; 1998.

37. McGuigan WM, Pratt CC. The predictive impact of domestic violence on three types of child maltreatment. Child Abuse Negl 2001;25(7):869–83.

38. Slep AMS, O'Leary SG. Parent and partner violence in families with young children: Rates, patterns, and connections. J Consult Clin Psychol 2005;73(3): 435–44.

39. Edleson JL. The overlap between child maltreatment and women battering. Violence Against Women 1999;5(2):134–54.
40. Rumm PD, Cummings P, Krauss MR, et al. Identified spouse abuse as a risk factor for child abuse. Child Abuse Negl 2000;24(11):1375–81.
41. Tajima EA. The relative importance of wife abuse as a risk factor for violence against children. Child Abuse Negl 2000;24(11):1383–98.
42. Osofsky J. The impact of violence on children. Future Child 1999;9(3):33–49.
43. Zeanah CH, Scheeringa MS. The experiences and effect of violence in infancy. In: Osofsky J, editor. Children in a violent society. New York: Guilford; 1997. p. 97–123.
44. Jaffe PG, Wolfe D, Wilson S. Children of battered women. Newbury Park (CA): Sage; 1990.
45. Martin SG. Children exposed to domestic violence: psychological considerations for health care practitioners. Holist Nurs Pract 2002;16(3):7–15.
46. Hughes HM, Graham-Bermann SA, Gruber G. Resilience in children exposed to domestic violence. In: Graham-Bermann SA, Edleson JL, editors. Domestic violence in the lives of children: the future of research, intervention, and social policy. Washington, DC: American Psychological Association; 2001. p. 67–90.
47. Wolfe DA, Jaffe PG. Prevention of domestic violence: emerging initiatives. In: Graham-Bermann SA, Edleson JL, editors. Domestic violence in the lives of children: the future of research, intervention, and social policy. Washington, DC: American Psychological Association; 2001. p. 283–98.
48. Christian CW, Scribano P, Seidl T, et al. Pediatric injury resulting from family violence. Pediatrics 1997;99(2):E8.
49. Child Welfare Information Gateway. Child protection in families experiencing domestic violence. Washington, DC: U.S. Department of Health and Human Services, Children's Bureau; 2003. Available at: https://www.childwelfare.gov/pubPDFs/domesticviolence.pdf.
50. Zeanah CH, Scheeringa M. Evaluation of posttraumatic symptomatology in infants and young children exposed to violence. In: Osofsky JD, Fenichel E, editors. Islands of safety: assessing and treating young victims of violence. Washington, DC: Zero Three; 1996. p. 9–14.
51. Osofsky JD. Children who witness domestic violence: the invisible victims. Soc Policy Rep 1995;9(3):1–20.
52. Rossman BBR. Longer term effects of children's exposure to domestic violence. In: Graham-Bermann SA, Edleson JL, editors. Domestic violence in the lives of children: the future of research, intervention, and social policy. Washington, DC: American Psychological Association; 2001. p. 35–65.
53. Christie D, Viner R. Adolescent development. BMJ 2005;330:301–4.
54. Hughes HM. Psychological and behavioral correlates of family violence in child witness and victims. Am J Orthop 1988;58(1):77–90.
55. Flaherty E, Stirling J. The Committee on Child Abuse and Neglect. The pediatrician's role in child maltreatment prevention. Pediatrics 2010;126(4):833–41.
56. Institute of Medicine. Clinical preventive services for women: Closing the gaps. Washington, DC: The National Academies Press; 2011.
57. Feder G, Ramsay J, Dunne D, et al. How far does screening women for domestic (partner) violence in different health-care settings meet criteria for a screening programme? systematic reviews of nine UK national screening committee criteria. Health Technol Assess 2009;13(16):iii–347.
58. Rabin RF, Jennings JM, Campbell JC, et al. Intimate partner violence screening tools: a systematic review. Am J Prev Med 2009;36(5):439–45.e4.

59. Domestic Intimate Partner Violence. AAP.org. Available at: http://www.aap.org/en-us/advocacy-and-policy/aap-health-initiatives/resilience/Pages/Domestic-Intimate-Partner-Violence.aspx. Accessed August 4, 2020.

60. Thackeray JD, Hibbard R, Dowd MD, et al. Intimate partner violence: the role of the pediatrician. Pediatrics 2010;125(5):1094–100.

61. Groves B, Augustyn M, Lee D, et al. Identifying and responding to domestic violence: consensus recommendations for pediatric and adolescent health. San Francisco: The Family Violence Prevention Fund; 2004.

62. Bressler C, Brink FW, Crichton KG. Screening for Intimate Partner Violence in the Pediatric Emergency Department. Clin Pediatr Emerg Med 2016;17(4):249–54.

63. Peterman A, Potts A, O'Donnell K, et al. Pandemics and violence against women and children. CGD Working Paper 528. Washington, DC: Center for Global Development; 2020.

64. Rempel E, Donelle L, Hall J, et al. Intimate partner violence: a review of online interventions. Inform Health Soc Care 2019;44(2):204–9.

65. Ford-Gilboe M, Varcoe C, Scott-Storey K, et al. A tailored online safety and health intervention for women experiencing intimate partner violence: the iCAN plan 4 safety randomized controlled trial protocol. BMC Public Health 2017;17(1):273.

66. van Gelder NE, van Rosmalen-Nooijens KAWL, Ligthart A, et al. SAFE: an eHealth intervention for women experiencing intimate partner violence – study protocol for a randomized controlled trial, process evaluation and open feasibility study. BMC Public Health 2020;20(1):640.

67. Wood SN, Glass N, Decker MR. An integrative review of safety strategies for women experiencing intimate partner violence in low- and middle-income countries. Trauma Violence Abuse 2021;22(1):68–82.

Executions and Police Conflicts Involving Children, Adolescents and Young Adults

Tiffani J. Johnson, MD, MSc[a],*, Joseph L. Wright, MD, MPH[b]

KEYWORDS

- Police violence • Policing • Race • Racism • Disparities • Discrimination
- Implicit bias

KEY POINTS

- Police executions represent an urgent public health crisis and have become a leading cause of death among young Black males in the United States.
- Beyond executions, harmful treatment and excessive use of force by police disproportionately impact children, adolescents, and young adults of color.
- Although less publicized, young Black girls, adolescents, and young women have also been overpoliced while underprotected, particularly in the education setting.
- Executions and conflicts inflicted by police have negative impacts on youth academic, mental health, and physical health outcomes.
- Pediatricians and other health care providers must recognize police violence as a public health crisis, and act through clinical practice, education, advocacy, and research.

INTRODUCTION

The oppression of communities of color by law enforcement has received heightened attention, not only in the public discourse, but also among health care providers and organized medicine.[2–4] This has been particularly evident since the executions of Eric Garner, Michael Brown, and Tamir Rice by police in 2014; and more recently, the national awakening regarding anti-Black police violence sparked by the executions of George Floyd and Breonna Taylor in 2020.[5,6] These tragic events have been brought to light in the setting of an increased use of police body cameras and widespread

Author note: Following the convention of the Associated Press, the authors have capitalized the word Black but not white when used in the context of race and culture.[1]
a Department of Emergency Medicine, University of California, Davis School of Medicine, 4150 V Street Suite 2100, Sacramento, CA 95817, USA; b Pediatrics and Health Policy & Management, University of Maryland Schools of Medicine and Public Health, University of Maryland Capital Region Health, 3001 Hospital Drive, Executive Suite, Cheverly, MD 20785, USA
* Corresponding author.
E-mail address: tjo@ucdavis.edu

Pediatr Clin N Am 68 (2021) 465–487
https://doi.org/10.1016/j.pcl.2020.12.012
0031-3955/21/© 2020 Elsevier Inc. All rights reserved.

pediatric.theclinics.com

access to cell phone recordings by citizens capturing some of the appalling and gruesome acts at the hands of law enforcement. With the backdrop of the coronavirus disease-2019 global pandemic with devastating ethnic and racial disparities, national attention regarding the impact of anti-Black police violence has been further sustained by the 24-hour news cycle, social media, and powerful protests. It is imperative that pediatricians are equipped to provide anticipatory guidance to patients and families, and engage in meaningful steps to address police violence as a public health crisis.

This article provides a state-of-the-science overview of executions and police conflicts involving children, adolescents, and young adults. It begins by describing the more recent epidemiology with a focus on the period between 2014 and 2020. The article then provides an overview of the centuries-long history of white supremacy and anti-Black racism as a foundation of modern-day policing, from slave patrols in the 1700s, to the modern-day war on drugs that has been described as the "new Jim Crow." The article then examines the social determinants of the inequities in juvenile contact and conflict with police, exploring how age, race, gender, class, and geography impact police encounters. Next, we provide evidence of the impact of adverse policing on youth academic, mental health, and physical health outcomes. The article concludes with suggested strategies for pediatricians and public health professionals to help address police violence as a public health crisis through clinical practice, education, advocacy, and research. As pediatric providers who are committed to mitigating the impact of violence on children in all its forms, it is important to acknowledge and take steps to protect the rights of children to live free of violence and trauma enacted by law enforcement.

EPIDEMIOLOGY OF POLICE CONFLICTS INVOLVING YOUTH

The true prevalence of police-related deaths is difficult to determine owing to underreporting in official databases, with a lack of federal requirements for reporting and inconsistent state requirements.[7] However, with the increase use of novel data sources, researchers are providing evidence that being killed by the police is a leading cause of death of young Black males in the United States, representing a major health inequity that must be urgently addressed.[8,9] For example, using data from the National Vital Statistics System on deaths including codes for legal encounters, researchers have estimated that Black men and boys face a lifetime risk of being killed by the police of 1 in 1000 in comparison with a risk of 39 per 100,000 for white men and boys.[8] Data from Fatal Encounters, an independent source of data on police-involved deaths, found that the risk of being killed by the police was 3.2 to 3.5 times higher for Black men and 1.4 to 1.7 times higher for Latino men in comparison with white men.[10] News reports of high-profile police shootings also provide important insights into the epidemiology of police executions of youth. Data from the *Washington Post* on police fatal shootings gathered from local news reports since 2015 indicates unarmed Black men are 4 times as likely to be killed by police than unarmed white men.[11]

Individuals with untreated mental illness are also more likely to be killed by law enforcement.[12] For example, Salt Lake City police shot and killed 13-year-old Linden Cameron after his mother called 911 seeking help while he was having a mental health crisis.[13,14] Twenty-nine-year-old Osaze Osagie met a similar fate when his father called the police requesting a mental health check after he sent a text message threatening to kill himself.[15] These examples speak to how ill-equipped law enforcement is to properly respond to mental health crises, often causing harm when they are called on for help.

Those with mental illness also experience harm by the police even while seeking treatment in the health care system. For example, 26-year-old Alan Pean presented to a hospital for symptoms including agitation and delusions. However, after crashing his car on arrival he was admitted to a surgical floor for observation. When his unaddressed mental health symptoms escalated, armed hospital security were called and they shocked the patient with a Taser, shot him in the chest, and placed him in handcuffs.[16] In a similar case, Jonathan Warner was shot and critically injured by hospital security after he became agitated by the potential for an involuntary psychiatric hold.[17] In Ohio, a man brought to the emergency department by police for psychiatric illness became violent and was shot in the neck by an armed security officer.[18] These cases highlight the importance of hospital policies and staff training to de-escalate and manage behavioral health issues without the use of weapons.

Armed law enforcement officers from the community have also caused harm in the health care setting, with one Los Angeles emergency department experiencing 2 police-involved patient shootings in the past 5 years. In 2015, 26-year-old Ruben Jose Herrera, who had a history of bipolar disorder, was executed while in police custody after allegedly reaching for the officers' guns. In October 2020, an agitated patient being treated for a psychiatric condition was shot and critically wounded by a deputy who was guarding another patient's room.[19]

Beyond the disturbing statistics of police related deaths, as pediatricians we must recognize these children and adolescents as our patients, such as 17-year-old Antwon Rose, a passenger in a car stopped by the police who was shot as he ran away from the scene unarmed.[20] We must honor these lives taken as sons and daughters, sisters and brothers, in some cases mothers and fathers. We must acknowledge the dreams and potential unrealized, such as Treyvon Martin, who had dreams of becoming a pilot before being killed at the age of 17 by a neighborhood watch volunteer while walking home; or Breonna Taylor, the 26-year-old emergency medical technician and aspiring nurse, who was shot to death while in her bed by police serving a search warrant related to a narcotics investigation of her ex-boyfriend, who was already in custody at the time.[6] After her death, a grand jury indicted 1 officer for "wanton endangerment," not for the shots that killed her, but for the 10 shots fired that missed her and passed into a neighbor's apartment. No charges have been filed for her death. It is important that we say their names. Although there are too many to recount in this text, we list some of the unarmed Black children, adolescents, and young adults under 30 years old killed by police, acknowledging that this list is not comprehensive and there are others who remain uncounted (**Table 1**). It is also important to acknowledge that, even among those killed while reportedly armed with a weapon, police reports of weapons and imminent threat are often contradicted by witness reports.[21] Furthermore, their executions are juxtaposed to numerous armed white mass shooters who police safely apprehended without incident.[22]

In addition to fatal shootings, the excessive use of force and other acts of violence also occur when children, adolescents, and young adults come into contact with the police. One example is the intentionally reckless ride experienced by a handcuffed, and otherwise unrestrained, Freddie Gray in the back of a Baltimore police paddy wagon that ultimately broke his neck. Another example involved the medical profession being complicit with police excessive use of force against 23-year-old Elijah McClain. He was walking home from the store unarmed and committing no crime other than being young, black, male, and "different," when 911 was called because he was wearing a ski mask and looked suspicious. During the ensuing conflict with the police, he pleads: "I was just going home. I'm an introvert and I'm different… I'm just different. I'm just different. That's all. I'm so sorry. I have no gun. I don't do

Table 1
Say their names: Unarmed black children, adolescents, and adults under 30 executed by police[a]

Name	Age	Location	Date
Deontae Keller	20	Portland, OR	May 1996
Amadou Diallo	22	Bronx, NY	Mar 1999
Kendra James	21	North Portland, OR	May 2003
James Brisette	17	New Orleans, LA	Sept 2005
Sean Bell	23	Queens, NY	Nov 2006
Tarika Wilson	26	Lima, OH	Jan 2008
Oscar Grant	22	Oakland, CA	Jan 2009
Aaron Campbell	25	Portland, OR	Jan 2010
Aiyana Stanley-Jones	7	Detroit, MI	May 2010
Rekia Boyd	22	Chicago, IL	Mar 2012
Shantel Davis	23	Brooklyn, NY	Jun 2012
Shelly Frey	27	Houston, TX	Dec 2012
John Crawford III	22	Dayton, OH	Aug 2014
Michael Brown	18	Ferguson, MO	Aug 2014
Tamir Rice	12	Cleveland, OH	Nov 2014
Akai Gurley	28	Brooklyn, NY	Nov 2014
Ezell Ford	25	Florence, CA	Aug 2014
Jeremy Lett	28	Tallahassee, FL	Feb 2015
Lavall Hall	25	Miami Gardens, FL	Feb 2015
Tony Robinson	19	Madison, WI	Mar 2015
Anthony Hill	27	Atlanta, GA	Mar 2015
Brandon Jones	18	Cleveland, OH	Mar 2015
Freddie Gray	25	Baltimore, MD	Apr 2015
William Chapman	18	Portsmith, VA	Apr 2015
David Felix	24	New York City, NY	Apr 2015
Brendon Glenn	29	Venice, CA	May 2015
Kris Jackson	22	South Lake Tahoe, CA	June 2015
Victor Larosa	23	Jacksonville, FL	Jul 2015
Darrius Stewart	19	Memphis, TN	Jul 2015
Albert Davis	23	Orlando, FL	Jul 2015
Christian Taylor	19	Arlington, TX	Aug 2015
Keith McLeod	19	Reisterstown, MD	Sept 2015
Anthony Ashford	29	Point Loma, CA	Oct 2015
Jamar Clark	24	Minneapolis, MN	Nov 2015
Nathaniel Harris Pickett	29	Barstow, CA	Nov 2015
Keith Childress	23	Las Vegas, NV	Dec 2015
Calin Roquemore	24	Beckville, TX	Feb 2016
Dyzhawn Perkins	19	Arvonia, VA	Feb 2016
David Joseph	17	Austin, TX	Feb 2016
Christopher Davis	21	East Troy, WI	Feb 2016
Jessica Nelson-Williams	29	San Francisco, CA	May 2016

(continued on next page)

Table 1
(continued)

Name	Age	Location	Date
Michael Wilson	27	Hallandale Beach, FL	May 2016
Vernell Bing	22	Jacksonville, Fl	May 2016
Deravis Rogers	22	Atlanta, GA	Jun 2016
Dalvin Hollins	29	Tempe, AZ	Jul 2016
Donnell Thompson	27	Compton, CA	Jul 2016
Levonia Riggins	22	Tampa, FL	Aug 2016
Darrion Barnhill	23	Reagan, TN	Jan 2017
Chad Robertson	25	Chicago, IL	Feb 2017
Raynard Burton	19	Detroit, MI	Feb 2017
Alteria Woods	21	Gifford, FL	Mar 2017
Jordan Edwards	15	Balch Springs, TX	Apr 2017
Ricci Holden	24	Converse, LA	May 2017
Dejuan Guillory	27	Mamou, LA	Jul 2017
Isaiah Tucker	28	Oshkosh, WI	Jul 2017
Anthony Ford	27	Miami, FL	Aug 2017
Calvin Toney	24	Baton Rouge, LA	Nov 2017
Darion Baker	22	Stratford, TX	Feb 2018
Stephon Clark	23	Sacramento, CA	Mar 2018
Cameron Hall	27	Casa Grande, AZ	Mar 2018
Juan Jones	25	Danville,VA	Apr 2018
Marcus-Davis Peters	24	Richmond, VA	May 2018
Antwon Rose II	17	Pittsburgh, PA	Jun 2018
Jalon Johnson	17	Houston, TX	Aug 2018
O'Shae Terry	24	Arlington, TX	Sept 2018
James Leatherwood	23	Hollywood, FL	Sept 2018
Botham Jean	26	Dallas, TX	Sept 2018
Jacob Servais	29	Vineland, NJ	Oct 2018
Charles Roundtree	18	San Antonio, TX	Oct 2018
Danny Washington	27	Franklin Twshp, PA	Dec 2018
Jimmy Atchison	21	Atlanta, GA	Jan 2019
Isaiah Lewis	17	Edmond, OK	Apr 2019
Elijah McClain	23	Aurora, Colorado	Aug 2019
Atatiana Jefferson	28	Fort Worth, TX	Oct 2019
Michael Dean	28	Temple, TX	Dec 2019
Jaquyn Light	20	Graham, NC	Jan 2020
Breonna Taylor	26	Louisville, KY	Mar 2020
Barry Gedeus	27	Ft. Lauderdale, FL	Mar 2020
Shaun Fuhr	24	Seattle, WA	May 2020
Maurice Gordon	28	Bass River, NJ	May 2020

Owing to inconsistencies in data collection, this table does not represent a comprehensive list.
 [a] Data sources include: https://www.cnn.com/2015/04/05/us/controversial-police-encounters-fast-facts/index.html; https://www.bbc.com/news/world-us-canada-52905408; https://www.buzz feednews.com/article/nicholasquah/heres-a-timeline-of-unarmed-black-men-killed-by-police-over; https://www.washingtonpost.com/graphics/investigations/police-shootings-database/; and https:// www.koin.com/news/special-reports/a-brief-history-of-african-americans-killed-by-ppb/.

that stuff. I don't do any fighting. Why are you attacking me?"[23] Officers threatened to assault him with a Taser and police dog, and placed him in a carotid hold twice resulting in loss of consciousness, vomiting, and difficulty breathing. When emergency medical services was called, Elijah who weighed 140 pounds (less than 65 kg) and was already on the ground physically restrained in handcuffs, was then chemically restrained with 500 mg of ketamine (more than 1.5 times the 5 mg/kg protocol dose based on an incorrectly estimated weight of 100 kg). He suffered a cardiac arrest and was later declared brain dead before being taken off of life support.[24] This use of ketamine for law enforcement purposes does not represent an isolated incident. According to a 2018 Minneapolis police conduct review, mentions of the use of ketamine on detainees in police reports sharply increased from an average of 4 times per year before 2015 to 62 times in 2017. There was also clear documentation of police officer involvement in medical decision making regarding ketamine administration, including officers explicitly requesting ketamine administration.[25] Concerns about inappropriate ketamine use are further supported by a whistleblower lawsuit filed by a former Minnesota paramedic claiming being pressured by police to administer ketamine without medical indications.[26] The American Society of Anesthesiologists and the American College of Emergency Physicians have issued a joint statement to "firmly oppose the use of ketamine or any other sedative/hypnotic agent to chemically incapacitate someone solely for a law enforcement purpose and not for a legitimate medical reason."[27]

Police conflicts also come in the form of dog attacks, use of conducted electric weapons (eg, Tasers), and beatings. For example, excessive, avoidable, and disproportionate use of police dogs as weapons threatens the safety of children, adolescents, and young men of color. An investigation of the Ferguson Police Department revealed the use of dogs out of proportion to the level of threat being posed for nonviolent incidents and included canine injuries to children.[28] The investigation also revealed evident disparities, with the victim being Black in 100% of police canine incidents where race was recorded. Data from the Los Angeles County Police Department similarly revealed that from 2004 to 2012, 89% of police canine attacks were against Blacks and Latinos[29] and was reported as 100% the first 6 months of 2013.[30] Similar trends have been reported in St. Paul, where most of the people bitten by the canine unit were young Black males, the youngest being a 12-year-old boy.[31] Data from the National Electronic Injury Surveillance System indicates that of police dog bite injuries resulting in emergency department visits from 2005 to 2013, 18.8% involved children and adolescents under the age of 20 years, 42% were Black, and 95% were male.[32] Similar findings of disparities in use of force are seen for Tasers, with a study of 1 police department revealing that non-white subjects are nearly twice as likely to have a Taser used against them in comparison with white suspects, even after controlling for confounders, including level of resistance.[33]

There is also a growing body of quantitative and qualitative research documenting the experiences of violence inflicted by police. For example, a cross-sectional survey of adults in Baltimore and New York City, which included a subset of young adults age 18 to 24 years, reported experiences of police violence, including sexual violence, physical violence with and without a weapon, psychological violence, and neglect.[34] In this study, reports of experiencing police violence were higher among racial/ethnic and sexual minorities (those who identified as homosexual or transgender). In qualitative interviews with adolescents males ages 13 to 19 living in disadvantaged neighborhoods in St. Louis, Missouri, participants reported experiences of physical abuse during encounters with the police, including being shoved, punched, and kicked.[35] When looking at factors that contribute to police use of force, data based on ride along observer reports reveals that officers are more likely to use force with suspects who are male, non-white, poor, and younger, irrespective of the suspect's behavior.[36] Additional research shows higher levels of force on individuals with mental illness.[37] The literature on the impact of police officer demographics is mixed, and limitations in the available data make it difficult to draw meaningful conclusions about the role of racial discordance and police use of force.[38–40]

Adolescents and young adults have also been met with gratuitous violence from the police during protests, both historically as well as more recent times. Haunting photographs of Civil Rights demonstrations in the 1960s depict protesters being assaulted with fire hoses and police dogs as instruments of terror and oppression.[41] More recent protesters over the past decade have been met with militarized vehicles, chemical irritants (eg, tear gas, pepper spray), "less than lethal" kinetic impact projectiles (eg, beanbag rounds—small synthetic bags filled with lead pellets and fired from a shotgun, rubber bullets), and an overall unnecessary escalation and force for crowd dispersal.[42] For example, 20-year-old protester Joshua Howell sustained a skull fracture after being shot in the head by a beanbag round indiscriminately fired by officers into the crowd in response to another protester throwing a bottle of water.[43] There have been several reports of police-fired projectiles resulting in severe ocular injuries[44] and other forms of severe head and facial trauma.[45] Such aggressive use of force has ironically occurred during protests against anti-Black police violence. This militarized response by police to unarmed antiracism protesters stands in stark contrast to the lack of force toward coronavirus disease-2019 antilockdown protesters, even when those protesters, who were predominately white men, were heavily armed with assault weapons.[46]

Although most of the literature and media attention regarding police violence has focused on boys and young men of color, it is important to recognize the impact on girls and young women. This includes police executions of Black women with mental illness, as well as violence and aggression during traffic stops.[47,48] A notable proportion of women have also reported experiencing police victimization, including physical, sexual, and psychological violence, with significantly higher rates among women who are racial/ethnic minorities.[49]

Exposure to violence from police is not limited to the community, but also occurs at an alarming rate in the education system. For example, 2019 school video surveillance captured Chicago police officers dragging a 16-year-old girl down the stairs, and kicking, hitting, and tasing her.[50] The incident was provoked by the minor infraction of the teen having her phone out while in class and the incident was unnecessarily escalated by officers while she was being escorted out of the school. Similar excessive use of force was captured on video in a South Carolina school, where a school resource officer flipped the desk and dragged a student from the classroom after she refused to surrender her cell phone.[51] In addition to physical harm, research has also documented psychological violence from school resource officers (eg, humiliation, verbal abuse).[52] These examples help to illustrate the conflicts involving police that ensue when children of color are disproportionately criminalized for developmentally appropriate adolescent misbehaviors.

In addition to physical violence, non-white individuals also report widespread experiences of unfair and harmful treatment by police.[53–55] This treatment includes experiencing inequitable and unfair enforcement of the law, disrespectful interactions, and unwarranted and sometimes unlawful stops and searches, as well as threats.[53] For example, in a Nashville community-based sample, Blacks were more than 3 times more likely than whites to report personal and vicarious unfair treatment by police.[56] Urban youth also report being victimized by police harm in the form of verbal abuse (including racial slurs), abandonment in unfamiliar neighborhoods, and planted evidence. Although these experiences were most prominent among Black youth, they were also reported by white youth who associated with Black youth and those who spent time in Black or racially mixed neighborhoods. By contrast, little police contact was reported by white youth when in white neighborhoods. These findings demonstrate how both race and place impact youth interactions with the police.[35] Beyond citizen reports, analysis of officer-worn body camera footage reveals officers speaking with more disrespect during interactions with Black community members in comparison with white community members.[57] This footage helps to support the perceptions of discriminatory and disparaging interactions with police.

ROLE OF RACIAL BIAS

It is important to recognize and acknowledge the role of bias and stereotyping in the criminal justice system. For example, studies have demonstrated an implicit stereotypical association between Black race and crime.[58–60] This bias contributes to racial profiling and increased contact with the police. Such stereotypes are in part fueled by the media, with prior research showing that Blacks are over-represented as lawbreakers in the news in comparison with their crime rates, whereas whites are under-represented.[61] Exposure to the over-representation of Blacks as criminals on news programs is associated with perceptions of Blacks as violent among the general public.[62] Simulation studies also provide important insight into how implicit bias impacts decisions to shoot. In a meta-analysis published in 2015 of 42 simulation-based studies examining racial shooter biases, participants were quicker to shoot armed Black targets, slower to not shoot unarmed Black targets, and more likely to have a liberal shooting threshold for Black targets compared with white targets.[63]

Consistent with research demonstrating implicit bias against Black children in the health care setting,[64] implicit bias in the justice system is also not limited to adult populations. For example, in a study in which police officers were given an implicit dehumanization task, officers who implicitly associated Blacks with apes more frequently used force against Black children relative to children of other races throughout their career.[65] Other investigators have found that the implicit dehumanization of Blacks is associated with greater perceptions of Black males as a threat and greater use of deadly force.[66] The adultification of Black children and adolescents in the justice system is also worth noting, with Black and Latino juvenile felony suspects being perceived as being older than their actual age and more culpable.[65] This finding was also evident in the execution of Tamir Rice, when police were responding to a 911 call of someone in the park who was "probably a juvenile" with a gun that was "probably fake." Reports indicate Tamir, while holding a toy gun, was shot within 2 seconds of police arriving to the scene. When calling for assistance, police described this 12-year-old child as a "Black male, maybe 20." When his 14-year-old sister came running to his aid, she was tackled and placed in handcuffs.[67]

Evidence from recent investigations of police departments related to highly publicized shootings offers additional evidence of the role of bias and overt discrimination. For example, the US Department of Justice investigation of the Ferguson Police Department concluded that:

> *disproportionate burden on African Americans cannot be explained by any difference in the rate at which people of different races violate the law. Rather, our investigation has revealed that these disparities occur, at least in part, because of unlawful bias against and stereotypes about African Americans. We have found*

substantial evidence of racial bias among police and court staff in Ferguson. For example, we discovered emails circulated by police supervisors and court staff that stereotype racial minorities as criminals, including one email that joked about an abortion by an African-American woman being a means of crime control.[28]

STRUCTURAL RACISM: HISTORICAL AND CONTEMPORARY CONTEXT

Although the role of personally mediated bias and stereotyping is important, it is also important to recognize that anti-Black police violence has deep-seated structural roots in the origins of policing. The historical and more contemporary context of structural racism exists in the form of policies, laws, and regulations that unfairly disadvantage certain individuals while unfairly advantaging others.[68] This background is important to provide a contextual framework of structural racism that partially explains the increased contact with law enforcement among communities of color that has harmful and sometimes deadly consequences for children, adolescents, and young adults that are both avoidable and unjust.

Slave Patrols of the South, Social Order in the North, and the Origins of Policing

Some of the earliest police forces in America were the slave patrols of the early 1700s, created in the South as a way to preserve the subjugation of Blacks in slavery and uphold white supremacy.[69–72] Their responsibilities included checking documents, regulating the movement of Blacks (enslaved and free), enforcing slave codes, monitoring gatherings of Blacks to guard against slave uprisings, and capturing runaway slaves. Severe and brutal methods were commonly used by slave patrols, whose purpose included terrorizing slaves and upholding the institution of slavery. One example of an early colonial municipal police force was established in Charleston, South Carolina, in the 1740s. By the 1830s, the Charleston Police Department grew to 100 officers whose primary purpose was as a slave patrol and represented the largest item in the Charleston municipal budget.[73] Another example is the Texas Rangers, the first organized state police force established in 1835 to retrieve runaway slaves escaping to Mexico.[74]

The structures of racism were seen at the foundation of early policing, even beyond slavery in the South. The first public municipal police departments were organized in the North in the early to mid 1800s in cities such as Boston, New York, and Philadelphia. These police departments served to maintain control over social classes that were perceived as dangerous at the time, including Irish and German immigrants, free Blacks, and the poor. Their function included enforcing laws targeting the poor related to alcohol and gambling, enforcing early laws minimizing the rights of Blacks, and suppressing labor strikes and hunger riots to maintain social order.[72]

Jim Crow, Sundown Towns, and Black Codes

Well into the mid to late twentieth century, police were also responsible for enforcing racist community laws and ordinances. For example, many municipalities had regulations limiting when Black people could freely move in town, with formal or informal policies that they had to leave before the sun went down. In these so-called sundown towns, punishment for violating these rules were enforced by police and often violent.[75,76]

Another example of early structural racism in policing includes a series of laws collectively known as "Black Codes." This code included vagrancy laws that were used almost exclusively to fine or incarcerate Black people who could not prove on demand and in writing that they were employed.[75] Once arrested and convicted, Black people were no longer protected by the Thirteenth Amendment, which prohibited slavery except as a punishment for crime. The labor of legally enslaved prisoners was often leased to private citizens, thereby generating considerable revenue for states, and further incentivizing arrests, predominately among Black populations.

Police Deputized and Sanctioned Vigilantism

With the ultimate failure of Reconstruction at the end of the 19th century to protect the physical safety and well-being of previously enslaved people and their descendants, the rise of the Ku Klux Klan and rampant vigilantism flourished. The unlawful killing of thousands of American descendants of slavery ensued, often by lynching, throughout the entirety of the Jim Crow period. In the absence of any meaningful political will to intercede at the federal, state, and particularly local levels, authorities were openly complicit in the enforcement of the continued subjugation and terrorism exacted against American descendants of slavery for fully a century after the end of the Civil War.

Perhaps the most notorious vigilante killing during this period involved an adolescent, 14-year-old Emmett Till from Chicago, who was lynched in Money, Mississippi, while visiting his uncle in the summer of 1955. Till's murder and his mother's brave advocacy in its aftermath insisting on an open casket at the teenager's funeral brought national awareness to ongoing oppression of Blacks and helped to galvanize the civil rights movement.[77] Emmett Till's story is just one of many examples of vigilantism sparked by rumors of Black males harming white females. Another event that was nearly erased in history was the Tulsa Race Riot of 1921.[78] The riot was precipitated when a Black man was accused of assaulting a 17-year-old white girl in an elevator in an office building. A lynch mob gathered at the courthouse, but was then met by Black war veterans to stop the lynching. When a riot erupted, several hundred white men from the lynch mob were then deputized by the police. The police-sanctioned violence that ensued included destruction of more than 1000 buildings that were burned, bombed, or looted, as well as the murder of hundreds of Black men, women, and children.

In more recent times, armed militias and vigilantes have had a growing presence at protests under the pretense of protecting businesses and property.[79] This includes 17-year-old Kyle Rittenhouse, who was accused of killing 2 people and injuring a third when he opened fire at a Kenosha, Wisconsin, protest over the police shooting of Jacob Blake, a 29-year-old Black man, in the back in the presence of his 3 children. Video footage seems to show police officers thanking armed vigilantes for their presence at the protest shortly before the shooting. Additional footage shows Rittenhouse walking from the scene of the shooting past officers unapprehended and still holding his weapon.[80] This tacit approval for vigilantes to protect property stands in stark juxtaposition to the failure to value and protect the lives and safety of Black children, adolescents, and young adults. The deaths of 17-year-old Trayvon Martin in 2012 and 25-year-old Ahmaud Arbery in 2020 are additional examples of vigilante executions of young Black males owing to racial stereotypes; both were suspected of crimes, chased, provoked into a conflict, and then executed under the thin veil of self-defense.[81]

The Civil Rights Movement, the War on Crime, and the War on Drugs

The 1960s witnessed a period of civil disobedience and peaceful protests against the oppression of Blacks in America. These demonstrations were often met with gratuitous violence from the police against peaceful protesters, including teens.[41] Civil rights protests also led to increased militarization of the police in the form of Special Weapons and Tactics teams.[72] Several well-known riots of the civil rights era, including those in Atlanta, Harlem, and San Francisco, were all in response to shootings of Black teenagers by white police officers.[82] The civil unrest that ensued led to a "War on Crime" declared by President Johnson, increasing police presence in predominately Black communities.[75]

In the 1970s, President Nixon identified drug abuse as public enemy number one and declared a "War on Drugs," resulting in increased federal funding to drug control agencies and mandatory sentencing for drug crimes. This War on Drugs was expanded in the 1980s in ways that disproportionately impacted communities of color. For example, minimum mandatory sentences were imposed for the possession of 5 g of crack cocaine, which was more commonly used in Black and Hispanic communities. In contrast, possession of 500 g of powder cocaine, which was more prevalent in white communities, was required for similar minimum sentencing.[83] This criminalization of substance abuse resulted in increased contact with police, and stands in stark contrasts with the more recent opioid abuse epidemic, predominantly impacting white and suburban communities, which has been addressed as a public health crisis.[84] Furthermore, as we see the decriminalization of marijuana in states across the country, the continued criminal justice approach to marijuana possession in juveniles must also be addressed to decrease youth contact with police caused by disparities in marijuana arrests.[85]

Beyond drug laws, there are other ways in which we continue to see the codification of structural racism in the criminal justice system. For example, the "3 strikes" laws of the 1990s implemented mandatory life sentences for repeat offenders, leading to significant racial disparities in punishment in communities of color who have greater contact with police and the criminal justice system.[75] Aggressive police tactics inspired by the "broken windows" theory of crime that strictly enforces minor crimes and disorderly behavior have also had disproportionate impact on communities of color.[75,86] A prime example is the proactive policing policies in New York City beginning in the early 1990s, including "stop and frisk" where pedestrians could be stopped, questioned, and searched for weapons (frisked).[87,88] Data indicate significant disparities, with more than 80% of pedestrians who were stopped and frisked were Black or Latino.[89] Although 88% of pedestrians stopped were innocent, police use of force occurred in more than 20% of stops.[87,90] These policies also resulted in an increased number of minority youth, specifically, having contact with the criminal justice system.[91,92] More than one-half of the stop and frisks in New York City were concentrated among adolescents and young adults under the age of 25,[88] with similar trends seen with other proactive policing approaches in other major cities across the country.[75]

Another example of how racism continues to act at the structural level is through disciplinary policies and practices in schools that lead to criminalizing youth behaviors. For example, in 2020 police body camera footage captured a 6-year-old girl who suffers from sleep apnea begging for help and pleading for another chance as she was placed in restraints and arrested for hitting school employees.[89] She was then booked and charged with misdemeanor battery before the charges were dropped the following day. Numerous other accounts of children of color being arrested and facing criminal charges for minor infractions in school have been reported.[93] This is often referred to as the "school-to-prison pipeline" owing to the resultant increased contact with law enforcement that funnels youth into the criminal justice system.[94] Research has demonstrated the association between police presence in schools with higher arrest rates for students, with a stronger effect for Black students in comparison with white and Hispanic students.[95] In addition to the structures and policies in place, these disparities are also related to stereotypes and bias in disciplinary practices that have been documented in the education setting.[96,97] For example, urban schools with more poor, Black, and Hispanic students are more likely to respond to student misbehaviors in a punitive manner and less likely to use restorative justice practices.[98] Such punitive treatment that increases contact of youth with police also increases their chance of experiencing harm from police.

The lack of accountability seen when officers execute Black and Brown bodies is another manifestation of structural racism that further devalues the lives of children, adolescents, and young adults who have historically experienced marginalization and oppression in many forms.[99,100] It is also important to recognize that individuals who experience racial bias and structural racism can internalize those negative messages about their own self-worth, leading to hopelessness and engagement in high risk activities.[68]

This historical context helps to illustrate the origins of how US police forces were established to maintain social order, which has often included preserving structures of racism, white supremacy, anti-immigrant ordinances, and injustice for poor and marginalized populations. It also provides context that the modern-day observed inequities in police contact and use of force in communities of color is not the result of a broken system or "a few bad apples." Rather, it is a manifestation of a system built on white supremacy and structural racism doing exactly what it was intended to do—that is, maintain a racist and class-based social order that unfairly oppresses and disadvantages some while unfairly advantaging others. Although the importance of community safety and crime prevention should not be ignored, the impact of the war on crime, the war on drugs, 3 strikes laws, aggressive policing tactics, and law enforcement in public schools should all be viewed in the context of understanding how structural racism has contributed to residential segregation and concentrated disadvantage as root causes of crime rates.[101]

The fact that the legal order not only countenanced but sustained slavery, segregation, and discrimination for most of our nation's history - and the fact that the police were bound to uphold that order - set a pattern for police behavior and attitudes toward minority communities that has persisted until the present day. That pattern includes the idea that minorities have fewer civil rights, that the task of the police is to keep them under control, and that the police have little responsibility for protecting them from crime within their communities.[73]

IMPACT OF EXECUTIONS AND POLICE CONFLICTS ON THE HEALTH AND WELL-BEING OF CHILDREN, ADOLESCENTS AND YOUNG ADULTS

In addition to lives lost from police executions, there is a growing body of literature demonstrating that experiencing violence and harmful treatment from police, whether personally or vicariously, is associated with negative academic, behavioral, and health (both mental and physical) outcomes.

Academic Outcomes

The presence of law enforcement in school has important implications for youth academic outcomes. Funding for police in schools is associated with decreased high school graduation rates and college enrollment, with the greatest effect seen for low-income students and Black and Hispanic students.[102] The vicarious trauma of executions involving police in communities of color also has negative impacts on Black and Hispanic but not white or Asian urban public high school students. These effects include lower grade point averages, rates of high school completion, and rates of college enrollment.[103,104] Other investigators have similarly found that increased surges of neighborhood aggressive police surveillance was associated with reduced test scores in adolescents, particularly among Black boys age 13 to 15 years.[105] This evidence explains how racism in the form of adverse policing in communities of color represents one of the root causes of the academic achievement gap.[106]

Mental Health Outcomes

Experiencing police violence is also associated with adverse mental health outcomes including psychotic experiences, suicidal attempts, and suicidal ideation that were not explained by confounders such as adverse childhood experiences, criminal involvement, or experiencing other forms of interpersonal violence.[34] Other investigators have also found an association between police victimization and increased odds of psychotic experiences[107] and suicide[108] attempts, as well as an association between harmful treatment and mood and anxiety disorders,[109] particularly among young urban men of color. Worse mental health outcomes such as trauma and anxiety symptoms have also been reported among young men aged 18 to 26 who reported having more contact with police.[110] Living under constant surveillance in neighborhoods with stop and frisk policing has also been linked with psychological distress.[111] In the setting of recent highly publicized police killings, nationally representative data have also found that Black Americans who are exposed to police killings of unarmed Blacks in their state report poorer mental health.[112] Although there are fewer data in the adolescent population, qualitative data from focus groups with Black boys ages 14 to 18 around national police brutality and police shootings identified fearing for their lives as a common theme.[113] The authors highlight the importance of vicarious police violence as a child advocacy issue owing to the psychological damage it can cause.

Physical Health Outcomes

Although data regarding this outcome are limited in children or adolescents, research in adult populations has demonstrated an association between Black men who experience personal or vicarious harm from police with shorter telomere length.[56] This finding is important, because shortened telomeres have been linked with poor health outcomes, including cardiovascular disease, metabolic disorders, and all-cause mortality.[114] Research also reveals that living in neighborhoods with invasive policing in the form of greater frequencies of stop and frisk policies, particularly in inequitably surveilled areas, is associated with a higher prevalence of diabetes, high blood pressure, and asthma episodes, as well as a higher body weight index and overall poor health.[87,113] Exposure to police violence is also associated with hypervigilance[115] and the resulting chronic stress associated with chronic vigilance is associated with a greater waist circumference in comparison with those who do not report vicarious harm.[116] These findings of the health impacts of discriminatory practices involving police encounters are also aligned with the extensive research demonstrating the relationship between general experiences of racial bias and discrimination with poor emotional,[117] behavioral,[118] and health outcomes.[119]

Although fair and respectful police encounters can promote well-being and enhance relations between police and the community,[120] there is compelling evidence of the negative impacts of unjust overpolicing of communities of color. Although additional research is still needed to fully understand the impact of police violence on the well-being of children and adolescents, these studies highlight the importance of screening for both direct and vicarious harmful police interactions and their associated psychological distress.

THE ROLE OF THE PEDIATRICIAN

Health care providers must recognize that violence by police is a major public health crisis that has substantial impacts on children, adolescents, and young adults. Pediatricians can play an important role by providing anticipatory guidance to families of all races on talking to children about the trauma and harm inflicted by police, particularly in the context of anti-Black police violence and executions.[3] The American Academy of Pediatrics in their policy statement "The Impact of Racism, on Child and Adolescent Health" recommends assessing patients for the social determinants of health that are often associated with racism and connecting families with resources.[121] This point is important, given the role of structural racism and concentrated disadvantage as root causes of increased contact with police. Given the role of harmful police interactions on mental health outcomes, pediatricians should screen patients for both direct contact with the police or general oversurveillance in their communities and have "the talk" with patients about their legal rights, strategies to get home safely, and offer support.[122] Patients should also be assessed for depression, anxiety, psychological distress, and other adjustment reactions that can occur with direct and vicarious police trauma, with appropriate referrals to mental health services as needed. It is also important to include these topics in medical student and graduate medical education curricula to equip the next generation of pediatricians to adequately address police violence as a public health crisis.

Although providing psychosocial supports is important, it is also important to advocate for police and justice reform so children and adolescents can to live free of violence and trauma enacted by law enforcement. As experts on child and adolescent health, pediatricians can play an important role engaging community leaders and policy makers to advocate for local and federal policies that decrease unnecessary youth contact with police in the education system and in general society. Some examples include:

- Increasing community investment in social determinants of health (eg, housing, education, equitable economic development, and youth recreation) as well as mental health and public health as a strategy for increasing public safety and decreasing crime. This effort will require reimagining city and state budgets, with greater allocation toward social services and less toward armed forces.
- Crisis intervention team approaches to manage mental health emergencies and decrease contact and conflict with police.[123]
- Reform laws and policies that unfairly criminalize marginalized populations and contribute to increased contact with and harmful treatment by police.
- Diversion programs and other community-based alternatives to juvenile incarceration.[90]
- Policies around marijuana that promote social justice and equity, such as inclusive licensing and investing marijuana tax revenue into communities adversely impacted by the war on drugs.
- Antiracism and implicit bias training for police accompanied by broader systemic reforms and evaluation of the impact of these trainings.
- Clear prehospital and hospital protocols to prevent police interference in medical decisions and care, and maintain the central role of medical decisions to do no harm and protect patients from the use of chemical restraints for punitive or law enforcement purposes.
- Greater accountability for death, violence, and other harmful treatment by police. This includes expeditious investigation and prosecution of cases where police unjustly murder or cause harm to citizens.

In addition to advocacy efforts, academic pediatricians and public health scholars can also engage in research examining the impact of policy changes on decreasing disparities in police contact with youth. Research requires consistent, accurate, standardized, and more comprehensive data reporting for police-involved injuries and deaths by law enforcement agencies. Hospitals, including children's hospitals, can also consistently track visits for which harm is caused by law enforcement. More research is also needed that focuses on the impact of police violence specifically in pediatric populations, and involving community members in the development of solutions. Additionally, although the impact of police violence is most pronounced in communities of color, there is some literature indicating disproportionate impacts among those who identify as homosexual or transgender. More research is needed in this population, as well as additional research on the intersection of race, sexual orientation, disability, and other historically marginalized affinity groups. There is also a need for health care systems and youth-serving organizations who have security or police forces to examine their data for potential disparities in security involvement, and, when identified, develop strategies for keeping patients and staff safe without causing harm or activating trauma.

SUMMARY

There is increasing public consciousness regarding the impact of executions and police conflicts, particularly against Black and Brown communities, as an urgent public health crisis. Unfortunately, our nation's children, adolescents, and young adults are not protected from experiencing police violence either personally and/or vicariously. Young people experience harm from police where they live, being executed while in their homes while eating ice cream (Botham Jean), playing video games (Atatiana Jefferson), or sleeping in their own beds (Breonna Taylor). They experience harm from police where they learn through overpolicing and acts of police violence in schools. They experience harm from police where they play (eg, Tamir Rice) and for simply being "different" (eg, Elijah McClain). More generally, they experience harm from police through an overall disregard for their lives and infringement on their rights. As pediatric providers, protecting children from harm is our central professional duty. It is therefore important for pediatricians to screen for both direct and vicarious adverse police interactions and their associated negative academic, emotional health, and physical health outcomes. Pediatricians can also play an important role in providing anticipatory guidance on how to talk to children about racism and police violence. Beyond clinical practice, pediatricians can engage in education and research efforts, and advocate for policies that help dismantle structures in place that perpetuate police violence against children, adolescents, and young adults.

CLINICS CARE POINTS

- Anticipatory guidance
  - Provide anticipatory guidance to families of all races on talking to children and adolescents about the harm inflicted by police, particularly in the context of anti-Black police violence and executions.
  - "The Talk" should be a part of anticipatory guidance to help patients understand their legal rights, strategies to get home safely, and offer support if they have an encounter with law enforcement.
- Screening

○ Screen children, adolescents, and young adults for depression, anxiety, psychological distress, and other adjustment reactions that can occur with direct and vicarious police trauma, with appropriate referrals to mental health services as needed.

- Medical care
  ○ Care for children who experience physical injuries cause by police should also address the psychosocial impacts of adverse police contacts.
  ○ Pediatric providers, practices, and institutions should consistently track visit for which harm is caused by law enforcement.

- Advocacy
  ○ Engage community leaders and policy makers to advocate for local and federal policies that decrease unnecessary youth contact with police.
  ○ Critically examine health care system policies regarding security and community law enforcement presence with an equity and antiracism lens, with a goal of identifying strategies to keep staff and patients safe without causing harm or activating trauma.

- Common pitfalls to avoid
  ○ Failure to ask patients about experiences of direct and indirect contact with the police.
  ○ Being a silent bystander and failing to advocate for police and justice reform necessary for children and adolescents to live free of violence and trauma enacted by law enforcement.

DISCLOSURE

None.

REFERENCES

1. Bauder D. AP says it will capitalize Black but not white. AP News 2020. Available at: https://apnews.com/article/7e36c00c5af0436abc09e051261fff1f. Accessed October 3, 2020.
2. Howard J. Racism is a public health issue and 'police brutality must stop,' medical group says. 2020. Available at: https://www.cnn.com/2020/06/01/health/racism-public-health-issue-police-brutality-wellness-bn/index.html. Accessed September 1, 2020.
3. American academy of pediatrics condemns racism, offers advice for families for how to talk to their children. Itasca (IL): American Academy of Pediatrics; 2020. Available at: https://services.aap.org/en/news-room/news-releases/aap/2020/american-academy-of-pediatrics-condemns-racism-offers-advice-for-families-for-how-to-talk-to-their-children/.
4. Dreyer BP, Trent M, Anderson AT, et al. The Death of George Floyd: bending the arc of history toward justice for generations of children. Pediatrics 2020;146(3). https://doi.org/10.1542/peds.2020-009639.
5. 8 Minutes and 46 Seconds: how George Floyd was killed in police custody. The New York Times 2020. Available at: https://www.nytimes.com/2020/05/31/us/george-floyd- investigation.html. Accessed June 11, 2020.
6. Oppel R, Taylor D, Bogel-Burroughs N. What we know about Breonna Taylor's case and death. The New York Times 2020;2020. Available at: https://www.nytimes.com/article/breonna-taylor-police.html. Accessed September 25, 2020.
7. Krieger N, Chen JT, Waterman PD, et al. Police killings and police deaths are public health data and can be counted. PLoS Med 2015;12(12):e1001915.
8. Edwards F, Lee H, Esposito M. Risk of being killed by police use of force in the United States by age, race-ethnicity, and sex. Proc Natl Acad Sci U S A 2019;116(34):16793–8.

9. Brunson R, Miller J. Young black men and urban policing in the united states. Br J criminology 2005;46(4):613–40.

10. Edwards F, Esposito M, Lee H. Risk of police-involved deaths by race/ethnicity and place, Unites States, 2012-2018. Am J Public Health 2019;108(9):1241–8.

11. Fatal Force. The Washington Post Last updated Oct 2020. Available at: https://www.washingtonpost.com/graphics/investigations/police-shootings-database/. Accessed October 6, 2020.

12. Fuller D, Lamb H, Biasotti M, et al. Overlooked in the undercounted: the role of mental illness in fatal law enforcement encounters. Arlington, VA: Treatment Advocacy Center; 2015. Available at: https://www.treatmentadvocacycenter.org/key-issues/criminalization-of-mental-illness/2976-people-with-untreated-mental-illness-16-times-more-likely-to-be-killed-by-law-enforcement-.

13. Elfrink T. 'He's a small child': Utah police shot a 13-year-old boy with autism after his mother called 911 for help. The Washington Post 2020. Available at: https://www.washingtonpost.com/nation/2020/09/08/linden-cameron-utah-autistic-shooting/. Accessed October 5, 2020.

14. Lowery L, Kindy K, Alexander K, et al. Distraught people, deadly results: officers often lack the training to approach the mentally unstable, experts say. 2015 Jun 30. 2015. Available at: https://www.washingtonpost.com/sf/investigative/2015/06/30/distraught-people-deadly-results/?itid=lk_inline_manual_12. Accessed October 5, 2020.

15. Rafacz S. Remembering Osaze. State College Magazine 2020. Available at: https://www.statecollegemagazine.com/articles/remembering-osaze/. Accessed March 1, 2020.

16. Rosenthal E. When the Hospital Fires the Bullet. The New York Times 2016. Available at: https://www.nytimes.com/2016/02/14/us/hospital-guns-mental-health.html. Accessed November 11, 2016.

17. Family of man shot inside Lynchburg hospital releases statement. WSLS 10 News 2016. Available at: https://www.wsls.com/news/2016/01/14/family-of-man-shot-inside-lynchburg-hospital-releases-statement/. Accessed November 13, 2020.

18. Gallek E, Gallek P. D L. Police: man shot after taking security officer's Taser in hospital emergency room. Fox 8 News 2015;2015. Available at: https://fox8.com/news/police-man-shot-after-taking-security-officers-taser-in-hospital-emergency-room/. Accessed November 23, 2020.

19. Pinho F. Man in critical condition after being shot by sheriff's depity at Harbour-UCLA Medical Center. The Los Angeles Times 2020 Oct 7, 2020. Availablet at: https://www.latimes.com/california/story/2020-10-07/sheriff-shooting-harbor-ucla. Accessed November 13, 2020.

20. CNN. Controversial police encounters fast facts 2020. Available at: https://www.cnn.com/2015/04/05/us/controversial-police-encounters-fast-facts/index.html. Accessed October 3, 2020.

21. Brown M, Ray R, Summers E, et al. # SayHerName: a case study of intersectional social media activism. Ethnic Racial Stud 2017;40(11):1831–46.

22. Holley P. Did 'whiteness' save the life of the alleged Planned Parenthood shooter? The Wash Post 2015. Available at: https://www.washingtonpost.com/news/post-nation/wp/2015/11/28/did-white-privilege-keep-the-planned-parenthood-shooter-from-being-killed-by-police/. Accessed November 29, 2015.

23. NBC News Now. Minute-To-Minute Breakdown Leading Up To Elijah McClain's Deadly Stop. June 27, 2020. Available at: https://www.youtube.com/watch?v=dGlHMZQtO7U. Accessed November 13, 2020.

24. Tompkins L. Here's what you need to know about Elijah McClain's death. The New York Times 2020;2020. Available at: https://www.nytimes.com/article/who-was-elijah-mcclain.html. Accessed November 11, 2020.

25. Office of Police Conduct Review. MPD Involvement in Pre-Hospital Sedation. July 26, 2018. Available at: https://lims.minneapolismn.gov/Download/File/1389/Office%20of%20Police%20Conduct%20Review%20(OPCR)%20Pre-Hosptial%20Sedation%20Study%20Final%20Report.pdf Accessed November 11, 2020.

26. Varagur K. Minnesota Paramedic Speaks Out Against Police Use of Ketamine Injections. The Intercept 2020;2020. Available at: https://theintercept.com/2020/08/25/ketamine-police-use-minnesota/. Accessed November 11, 2020.

27. American Society of Anesthesiologists. ASA/ACEP Joint Statement on the Safe Use of Ketamine in Prehospital Care. Aug 26, 2020. Available at: https://www.asahq.org/about-asa/newsroom/news-releases/2020/08/asa-acep-joint-statement-on-the-safe-use-of-ketamine-in-prehospital-care. Accessed November 16, 2020.

28. Justice UDo. Investigation of the Ferguson police department. US Department of Justice; 2015.

29. Police Assessment Resource Center. 33rd Semiannual Report of Special Counsel. Los Angeles Country Sheriffs Departments. September, 2013. Available at: https://static1.squarespace.com/static/5498b74ce4b01fe317ef2575/t/54ad49ace4b05e7c18c21652/1420642732418/33rd+Semiannual+Report.pdf. Accessed October 9, 2020.

30. Riggs M. So far this Year, L.A. County Sheriff's dogs have only bitten people of color. Bloomberg CityLab; 2013. Available at: https://www.bloomberg.com/news/articles/2013-10-09/so-far-this-year-l-a-county-sheriff-s-dogs-have-only-bitten-people-of-color. Accessed October 9, 2020.

31. Choi J. Partner or weapon? Police K-9 bites raise questions of control. MPRNews 2018. Available at: https://www.mprnews.org/story/2018/07/20/police-k9-bites-instincts-handlers-control-minnesota. Accessed July 15, 2020.

32. Loder RT, Meixner C. The demographics of dog bites due to K-9 (legal intervention) in the United States. J Forensic Leg Med 2019;65:9–14.

33. Crow MS, Adrion B. Focal concerns and police use of force: examining the factors associated with Taser use. Police Q 2011;14(4):366–87.

34. DeVylder JE, Oh H, Nam B, et al. Prevalence, demographic variation and psychological correlates of exposure to police victimisation in four US cities. Epidemiol Psychiatr Sci 2017;26(5):466–77.

35. Brunson RK, Weitzer R. Police relations with black and white youths in different urban neighborhoods. Urban Aff Rev 2009;44(6):858–85.

36. Terrill W, Mastrofski SD. Situational and officer-based determinants of police coercion. Justice Q 2002;19(2):215–48.

37. Rossler MT, Terrill W. Mental illness, police use of force, and citizen injury. Police Q 2017;20(2):189–212.

38. Smith BQ, Holmes MD. Police use of excessive force in minority communities: a test of the minority threat, place, and community accountability hypotheses. Social Probl 2014;61(1):83–104.

39. McElvain JP, Kposowa AJ. Police Officer Characteristics and the Likelihood of Using Deadly Force. Crim Justice Behav 2008;35(4):505–21.

40. Knox D, Mummolo J. Making inferences about racial disparities in police violence. Proc Natl Acad Sci 2020;117(3):1261–2.

41. Trent S. Trump's warning that 'vicious dogs' would attack protesters conjured centuries of racial terror. The Washington Post 2020. Available at: https://www.

washingtonpost.com/history/2020/06/01/trump-vicious-dogs-protesters-civil-rights-slavery/. Accessed September 30, 2020.

42. Harrington A. Tanks and rubber bullets vs. pussy hats and high-fives: a comparative look at the 2014 Ferguson Uprising and the 2017 Women's March on Washington. Hastings Women's LJ 2020;31:101.

43. O'Kane C. Say their names": the list of people injured or killed in officer-involved incidents is still growing. CBS News; 2020. Available at: https://www.cbsnews.com/news/say-their-names-list-people-injured-killed-police-officer-involved-incidents/. Accessed June 8, 2020.

44. Coleman AL, Williams GA, Parke DW. Ophthalmology and "rubber bullets." Ophthalmology 2020;127(10):1287–8.

45. Morrar S, Yoon-Hendricks A. 18-year-old shot in face with rubber bullet at Sacramento protest, recovering at hospital. The Sacramento Bee. 2020. Available at: https://www.sacbee.com/news/local/article243142336.html. Accessed May 31, 2020.

46. Zhou L, Amaria K. These photos capture the Stark contrast in police response to the George Floyd protests and the anti-lockdown protests. Vox 2020. Available at: https://www.vox.com/2020/5/27/21271811/george-floyd-protests-minneapolis-lockdown-protests. Accessed May 27, 2020.

47. Jacobs MS. The violent state: black women's invisible struggle against police violence. Wm Mary J Women L 2017;24:39.

48. Crenshaw K, Ritchie A, Anspach R, et al. Say her name: Resisting police brutality against black women. New York: African American Policy Forum. Center for Intersectional and Social Policy Studies, Columbia Law School; 2015.

49. Fedina L, Backes BL, Jun H-J, et al. Police violence among women in four US cities. Prev Med 2018;106:150–6.

50. Miller R. 'It's tragic': video shows Chicago police officers hitting, dragging student down stairs. USA Today 2019. Available at: https://www.usatoday.com/story/news/nation/2019/04/12/video-chicago-police-hit-dragged-student-dnigma-howard-lawsuit-says/3450778002/. Accessed April 12, 2019.

51. Faussct R, Southall A. Video shows officer flipping student in South Carolina, prompting inquiry. The New York Times 2015. Available at: https://www.nytimes.com/2015/10/27/us/officers-classroom-fight-with-student-is-caught-on-video.html. Accessed October 26, 2015.

52. Merkwae A. Schooling the police: race, disability, and the conduct of school resource officers. Mich J Race L 2015;21:147.

53. Tyler TR, Wakslak CJ. Profiling and police legitimacy: procedural justice, attributions of motive, and acceptance of police authority. Criminology 2004;42(2):253–82.

54. Bjornstrom EE. Race-ethnicity, nativity, neighbourhood context and reports of unfair treatment by police. Ethnic racial Stud 2015;38(12):2019–36.

55. Weitzer R, Tuch SA, Skogan WG. Police–community relations in a majority-Black city. J Res Crime Delinquency 2008;45(4):398–428.

56. McFarland MJ, Taylor J, McFarland CA, et al. Perceived unfair treatment by police, race, and telomere length: a Nashville community-based sample of black and white men. J Health Soc Behav 2018;59(4):585–600.

57. Voigt R, Camp NP, Prabhakaran V, et al. Language from police body camera footage shows racial disparities in officer respect. Proc Natl Acad Sci 2017;114(25):6521–6.

58. Welch K. Black criminal stereotypes and racial profiling. J Contemp Crim Justice 2007;23(3):276–88.

59. Eberhardt JL, Goff PA, Purdie VJ, et al. Seeing black: race, crime, and visual processing. J Pers Soc Psychol 2004;87(6):876.

60. Payne BK. Prejudice and perception: the role of automatic and controlled processes in misperceiving a weapon. J Pers Soc Psychol 2001;81(2):181.

61. Dixon TL, Linz D. Overrepresentation and underrepresentation of African Americans and Latinos as lawbreakers on television news. J Commun 2000;50(2): 131–54.

62. Dixon TL. Crime news and racialized beliefs: understanding the relationship between local news viewing and perceptions of African Americans and crime. J Commun 2008;58(1):106–25.

63. Mekawi Y, Bresin K. Is the evidence from racial bias shooting task studies a smoking gun? Results from a meta-analysis. J Exp Soc Psychol 2015;61: 120–30.

64. Johnson TJ, Winger DG, Hickey RW, et al. Comparison of physician implicit racial bias toward adults versus children. Acad Pediatr 2017;17(2):120–6.

65. Goff PA, Jackson MC, Di Leone BAL, et al. The essence of innocence: consequences of dehumanizing Black children. J Pers Soc Psychol 2014;106(4):526.

66. Ellawala TI. Pulling the trigger: dehumanization of African Americans and police violence. Scholarly Undergraduate Res J Clark 2016;2(1):1.

67. Dewan S, Oppel R. In Tamir Rice Case, Many Errors by Cleveland Police, Then a Fatal One. The New York Times 2015. Available at: https://www.nytimes.com/2015/01/23/us/in-tamir-rice-shooting-in-cleveland-many-errors-by-police-then-a-fatal-one.html. Accessed October 3, 2020.

68. Jones CP. Confronting institutionalized racism. Phylon 2002;50:7–22.

69. Walker S. Popular justice: a history of American criminal justice. Mich Law Rev 1980;79:921.

70. Hawkins H, Thomas R. White policing of black populations: A history of race and social control in America. In: Cashmore E, McLauglin E, editors. Out of Order? Policing Black People. London: Routledge; 1991. p. 65–86.

71. Hadden SE. Slave patrols: law and violence in Virginia and the Carolinas. Cambridge, MA: Harvard University Press; 2001.

72. Barlow DE, Barlow MH. A political economy of community policing. Policing 1999;22:646–74.

73. Williams H, Murphy PV. The evolving strategy of police: a minority view. Washington, DC: US Department of Justice, Office of Justice Programs, National Institute of Justice; 1990.

74. Samora J, Bernal J, Pena A. Gunpowder justice: a reassessment of the Texas Rangers. Notre Dame, IN: University of Notre Dame Press Notre Dame, Ind.; 1979.

75. National Academies of Sciences E, Medicine. Proactive policing: effects on crime and communities. Washington, DC: National Academies Press; 2018.

76. Loewen JW. Sundown towns: a hidden dimension of racism in America. New York: New Press; 2005.

77. Harold C, DeLuca KM. Behold the corpse: violent images and the case of Emmett Till. Rhetoric Public Aff 2005;8(2):263–86.

78. Brophy AL. The Tulsa Race Riot of 1921 in the Oklahoma Supreme Court. Oklahoma Law Rev 2001;54:67.

79. Ali SS. Where protesters go, armed militias, vigilantes likely to follow with little to stop them. NBC News 2020;2020.

80. Bates J. Teen Gunman charged with 'intentional homicide' after 2 killed during police shooting protests in Kenosha 2020. Available at: https://time.com/5883707/kyle-rittenhouse-murder-kenosha-protest-shootings/. Accessed August 26, 2020.

81. Blow C. The killing of Ahmaud Arbery. The New York Times 2020. Available at: https://www.nytimes.com/2020/05/06/opinion/ahmaud-arbery-killing.html. Accessed May 15, 2020.

82. DiPasquale D, Glaeser EL. The Los Angeles riot and the economics of urban unrest. J Urban Econ 1998;43(1):52–78.

83. Tonry M, Melewski M. The malign effects of drug and crime control policies on black Americans. Crime Justice 2008;37(1):1–44.

84. Gostin LO, Hodge JG, Noe SA. Reframing the opioid epidemic as a national emergency. JAMA 2017;318(16):1539–40.

85. Banys P. Mitigation of marijuana-related legal harms to youth in California. J Psychoactive Drugs 2016;48(1):11–20.

86. Wilson JQ, Kelling GL. Broken windows. Atlantic monthly 1982;249(3):29-38.

87. Sewell AA, Jefferson KA. Collateral damage: the health effects of invasive police encounters in New York City. J Urban Health 2016;93(1):42–67.

88. Rice SK, White MD. Race, Ethnicity, and Policing: New and Essential Readings. New York: New York University Press; 2010.

89. NYCLU. NYC: stop-and-frisk down safety up 2015. Available at: https://www.nyclu.org/sites/default/files/publications/stopfrisk_briefer_FINAL_20151210.pdf. Accessed September 28, 2020.

90. Owen MC, Wallace SB. Advocacy and collaborative health care for justice-involved youth. Pediatrics 2020;146(1):e20201755.

91. Brame R, Turner MG, Paternoster R, et al. Cumulative prevalence of arrest from ages 8 to 23 in a national sample. Pediatrics 2012;129(1):21–7.

92. Hagan J, Shedd C, Payne MR. Race, ethnicity, and youth perceptions of criminal injustice. Am Soc Rev 2005;70(3):381–407.

93. Crenshaw K, Ocen P, Nanda J. Black girls matter: pushed out, overpoliced, and underprotected: Center for Intersectionality and Social Policy Studies. New York: Columbia University; 2015.

94. Wald J, Losen DJ. Defining and redirecting a school-to-prison pipeline. New Dir youth Dev 2003;2003(99):9–15.

95. Homer EM, Fisher BW. Police in schools and student arrest rates across the United States: examining differences by race, ethnicity, and gender. J Sch violence 2020;19(2):192–204.

96. Kunesh CE, Noltemeyer A. Understanding disciplinary disproportionality: stereotypes shape pre-service teachers' beliefs about black boys' behavior. Urban Education 2019;54(4):471–98.

97. Okonofua JA, Eberhardt JL. Two strikes: race and the disciplining of young students. Psychol Sci 2015;26(5):617–24.

98. ANN PAYNE A, Welch K. Modeling the effects of racial threat on punitive and restorative school discipline practices. Criminology 2010;48(4):1019–62.

99. Chaney C, Robertson RV. Armed and dangerous? An examination of fatal shootings of unarmed black people by police. J Pan Afr Stud 2015;8(4):45–78.

100. Patterson GT, Swan PG. Police shootings of unarmed African American males: a systematic review. J Hum Behav Soc Environ 2016;26(3–4):267–78.

101. Jacoby SF, Dong B, Beard JH, et al. The enduring impact of historical and structural racism on urban violence in Philadelphia. Social Sci Med 2018;199:87–95.

102. Weisburst EK. Patrolling public schools: the impact of funding for school police on student discipline and long-term education outcomes. J Policy Anal Manage 2019;38(2):338–65.

103. Ang D. The effects of police violence on inner-city students. The Quarterly Journal of Economics 2021;136(1):115–68.

104. Gershenson S, Hayes MS. Police shootings, civic unrest and student achievement: evidence from Ferguson. J Econ Geogr 2018;18(3):663–85.

105. Legewie J, Fagan J. Aggressive policing and the educational performance of minority youth. Am Soc Rev 2019;84(2):220–47.

106. Lee J. Racial and ethnic achievement gap trends: reversing the progress toward equity? Educ Res 2002;31(1):3–12.

107. DeVylder JE, Cogburn C, Oh HY, et al. Psychotic experiences in the context of police victimization: data from the survey of police–public encounters. Schizophrenia Bull 2017;43(5):993–1001.

108. DeVylder JE, Frey JJ, Cogburn CD, et al. Elevated prevalence of suicide attempts among victims of police violence in the USA. J Urban Health 2017; 94(5):629–36.

109. Oh H, DeVylder J, Hunt G. Effect of police training and accountability on the mental health of African American Adults. Am J Public Health 2017;107(10): 1588–90.

110. Geller A, Fagan J, Tyler T, et al. Aggressive policing and the mental health of young urban men. Am J Public Health 2014;104(12):2321–7.

111. Sewell AA, Jefferson KA, Lee H. Living under surveillance: gender, psychological distress, and stop-question-and-frisk policing in New York City. Social Sci Med 2016;159:1–13.

112. Bor J, Venkataramani AS, Williams DR, et al. Police killings and their spillover effects on the mental health of black Americans: a population-based, quasi-experimental study. Lancet 2018;392(10144):302–10.

113. Staggers-Hakim R. The nation's unprotected children and the ghost of Mike Brown, or the impact of national police killings on the health and social development of African American boys. J Hum Behav Soc Environ 2016;26(3–4):390–9.

114. Haycock PC, Heydon EE, Kaptoge S, et al. Leucocyte telomere length and risk of cardiovascular disease: systematic review and meta-analysis. BMJ 2014;349: g4227.

115. Smith NA, Voisin DR, Yang JP, et al. Keeping your guard up: hypervigilance among urban residents affected by community and police violence. Health Aff 2019;38(10):1662–9.

116. McFarland MJ, Taylor J, McFarland CA. Weighed down by discriminatory policing: perceived unfair treatment and black-white disparities in waist circumference. SSM-population health 2018;5:210–7.

117. Wong CA, Eccles JS, Sameroff A. The influence of ethnic discrimination and ethnic identification on African American adolescents' school and socioemotional adjustment. J Personal 2003;71(6):1197–232.

118. Simons RL, Chen Y-F, Stewart EA, et al. Incidents of discrimination and risk for delinquency: a longitudinal test of strain theory with an African American sample. Justice Q 2003;20(4):827–54.

119. Paradies Y. A systematic review of empirical research on self-reported racism and health. Int J Epidemiol 2006;35(4):888–901.

120. Tyler TR. Procedural justice, legitimacy, and the effective rule of law. Crime Justice 2003;30:283–357.

121. Trent M, Dooley DG, Dougé J. The impact of racism on child and adolescent health. Pediatrics 2019;144(2):e20191765.
122. Maroney T, Zuckerman B. "The Talk," physician version: special considerations for African American, male adolescents. Pediatrics 2018;141(2). https://doi.org/10.1542/peds.2017-1462.
123. Watson AC, Fulambarker AJ. The crisis intervention team model of police response to mental health crises: a primer for mental health practitioners. Best Pract Ment Health 2012;8(2):71.

Community-Engaged and Informed Violence Prevention Interventions

Shaelyn M. Cavanaugh, MPH[a], Charles C. Branas, PhD[b],
Margaret K. Formica, MSPH, PhD[a],*

KEYWORDS

- Youth violence • Community violence • Sexual abuse • Physical abuse • Neglect
- Bullying • Prevention

KEY POINTS

- Violence against children is a multifaceted problem that is mediated by risk factors within the surrounding environment.
- Different types of violence should be addressed specifically and within their local context.
- A key aspect of the prevention of violence against youth is the mobilization of adult bystanders, which is integrated into many community-engaged approaches.
- Historically, violence was addressed by reacting to it once it had occurred, but community-based interventions focus on prevention and adaptation of societal norms.
- The rigorous evaluation of community-based programs faces many challenges related to feasibility, study design, and long-term funding.

INTRODUCTION

The community-based prevention of morbidity and mortality originated with efforts to control communicable disease through sanitation, housing, and urban reform. Since then, public health approaches have been increasingly applied to the modern causes of morbidity and mortality. In 2012, a committee convened by the Institute of Medicine produced a framework outlining the assessment of community-based interventions. This committee identified 3 strengths of such interventions: (1) impacts are not dependent on access to health care, (2) they can "reach individuals at all levels of risk," and (3) they take into account that many risk factors are "shaped by conditions not under an individual's control." The committee states that, "improving health and preventing

[a] Department of Public Health and Preventive Medicine, SUNY Upstate Medical University, 750 East Adams Street, Syracuse, NY 13210, USA; [b] Department of Epidemiology, Columbia University, Mailman School of Public Health, 722 West 168th Street, Room 1508, New York, NY 10032, USA
* Corresponding author.
E-mail address: formicam@upstate.edu

Pediatr Clin N Am 68 (2021) 489–509
https://doi.org/10.1016/j.pcl.2020.12.007
0031-3955/21/© 2020 Elsevier Inc. All rights reserved.

disease does not solely occur in the patient's examination room; it also takes place in the community of patients and their families, friends and neighbors, employers, teachers, and storekeepers."[1]

Historically, initiatives addressing violence were largely reactive rather than preventive, and violence was seen as a problem of individuals that should be addressed through law enforcement. The integration of community-based interventions to address violence on a population scale is based on theoretic and empiric evidence that the predictors of violence transcend the individual. These interventions advocate for a collective and preventive approach, and have shown promise across many domains. In this discussion of community-engaged violence prevention strategies, we provide examples of specific interventions that were designed to address 4 types of violence toward children: physical abuse, sexual abuse, community violence, and bullying. For each intervention, we describe the strategy and then the program evaluation (summarized in **Table 1**). This list is not meant to be comprehensive of all community-based programs that have been developed to date, but an avenue to provide examples of community-engaged youth violence prevention programs that have been used and evaluated.

PHYSICAL ABUSE PREVENTION

Currently, the largest body of evidence for prevention of violence against children is related to child maltreatment, which encompasses both physical abuse and neglect. Historically, organized attempts at decreasing maltreatment targeted individual families and caregivers. However, as a growing body of evidence has shed light on the intricate interplay of the community environment and child welfare, the US Advisory Board on Child Abuse and Neglect issued a series of reports in the early 1990s outlining the importance of a community engaged strategy for addressing this issue.[2]

Garbarino and Sherman[3] published a study that illuminated the concept of social risk as it relates to child abuse. They compared 2 communities that were similar in terms of socioeconomic and demographic profiles, but had large discrepancies in rates of child maltreatment. There was a higher level of "social impoverishment" in the community with a higher rate of maltreatment. This concept of impoverishment encompassed a negative image of one's community, a smaller social network, and lower use of the neighborhood as a resource. The authors state that, "a family's own problems seem to be compounded rather than ameliorated by the neighborhood context."[3] Many subsequent studies[4–6] have also demonstrated this link between abuse rates and collective efficacy, social network reach, and overall community organization. For example, Coulton and colleagues[4] found substantial variation in rates of reported maltreatment between different census tracts, and concluded that "child maltreatment is but one manifestation of community social organization." They found that the strongest predictors of child maltreatment were poverty, unemployment, female-headed households, and a high childcare burden. The authors point to a macrostructural impact of the community on child maltreatment.[4] A cross-sectional study published in 2016 revealed that "neighborhoods higher in collective efficacy, intergenerational closure, and social networks" had a lower rate of neglect, as well as physical and sexual abuse.[5] Neighborhood factors, including poverty, are widely shown to be significant predictors of sexual and physical violence and neglect against children, but to different degrees, with child neglect and physical abuse most strongly associated with neighborhood poverty status.[6]

It is important to note that, although limited and with varied results, research suggests a possible role of implicit bias with respect to race, ethnicity, and social and

Table 1
Summary of select community-based violence prevention initiatives

Intervention	Type of Violence	Summary of Intervention	Evaluation Methods	Outcomes
Strong Communities	Physical abuse and neglect	Creation of a culture of responsibility for child safety with neighbor-to-neighbor support	Matched comparison for self-reported survey data, hospital admissions, CPS cases	Compared with matched population: More self-reported efficacy Fewer hospital admissions Fewer CPS cases
Triple P		Locally publicized, multitier educational programming for parenting skill acquisition	Random assignment of communities to intervention vs control group	Statistically significant lower rates of CPS cases Foster care placement Hospital or ED visits owing to abuse
Durham Family Initiative		Identification of risk factors for abuse, while enhancing community capacity and accessibility of resources to prevent abuse	Matched comparison analysis for household surveys, professional surveys, CPS cases, hospital admissions	Compared with matched population: Greater reduction in self-reported parental stressors Lower rates of professional-estimated child abuse Fewer maltreatment related diagnoses in hospital and ED Fewer CPS cases
Durham Connects		Component of the Durham Family Initiative, implements universal home nursing visitation for all families with newborns in Durham County	Random assignment of individual families to intervention vs control	Compared with control group: Fewer emergency medical care episodes Higher use of community resources Higher rate of self-reported positive parenting behaviors

(continued on next page)

Table 1
(continued)

Intervention	Type of Violence	Summary of Intervention	Evaluation Methods	Outcomes
Circles of Safety: Stop It Now!	Sexual abuse	Social marketing, media, and training/ education for adult bystanders within communities. Targets perpetrators of abuse, adults who suspect abuse, and organizations including foster care programs, athletic departments, and other community organizations. Also includes a confidential helpline for guidance and resources.	Surveys of training participants Helpline contact data	Improvement in bystander awareness, warning signs, and confidence in reporting abuse Helpline data suggests it is a valuable resource for prevention
Darkness to Light: Stewards of Children		Education of adult stakeholders in the prevention of CSA within their spheres of influence. Incorporates a formal training program that is, approved for continuing educational credit by several professional credentialing organizations. Targets all adults within their personal and/or professional spheres, including parents, childcare professionals, educators, social workers, nurses, and more.	Surveys of training participants Rates of CPS reports by training participants Matched comparison analysis of CPS cases Random assignment of child care professionals to intervention vs control groups	Improvement in knowledge about prevention, recognition, and actions to take regarding CSA among trainees Increased rates CPS reporting among training participants after the intervention compared with before the intervention Increased rates of CPS reporting among training participants compared with a matched comparison group Improvement in knowledge, attitudes, and preventative behaviors in intervention vs control group

(continued on next page)

Table 1
(*continued*)

Intervention	Type of Violence	Summary of Intervention	Evaluation Methods	Outcomes
Enough Abuse Campaign		Comprehensive outreach materials and educational curricula, including workshops and presentations for key community stakeholders.	Statewide CPS reports Statewide survey of adults Survey data of educational program participants Random assignment of educators into intervention vs control group	Decrease in substantiated reports of CSA in Massachusetts and increase in preventative attitudes of residents in Massachusetts after statewide implementation of the campaign Increase in knowledge and attitudes about preventing CSA in educational program participants Statistically significant higher knowledge of prevalence, behaviors, impacts, and responses to CSA in intervention vs control group
CeaseFire	Community violence	Uses the CureViolence method of reducing youth involvement in neighborhood violence, based on stopping the spread of violence as if it were a communicable disease. Reaches high-risk youth with community members who may have been previously involved in criminal violence themselves.	Matched comparison analysis of intervention group vs neighboring communities in city Surveys of program participants	Four of 7 neighborhoods showed decrease in overall gun violence compared with matched areas, and 4 communities had a decrease in intensity and size of "shooting hot spots" Overall mixed results between the communities on violent crime impact and gang-associated violence

(*continued on next page*)

	Table 1 (continued)			
Intervention	**Type of Violence**	**Summary of Intervention**	**Evaluation Methods**	**Outcomes**
		These individuals are trusted and can change the culture of violence, and communicate conflict resolution strategies.		Survey data suggested that target population was successfully reached, and that violence interrupters did succeed in diffusing conflicts that often lead to retaliatory violence
Safe Streets			Matched comparison analysis of intervention groups (and their spillover areas) vs neighboring communities in city	Overall mixed results, but demonstrated that in intervention areas and their "spillover" areas, there were fewer homicides and nonfatal shootings.
			Surveys of program participants	Survey data suggested that outreach workers were successful avenues for youth to be connected with resources and opportunities, and hundreds of disputes were mediated, many of these disputes involved guns.
Save Our Streets			Matched comparison analysis of intervention group vs neighboring communities in city	Decrease in shooting rates in intervention areas, with a corresponding increase in rates in matched comparison areas
			Surveys of community members	Survey of community members revealed an overall high awareness of the program and a high confidence in the program

(continued on next page)

Table 1 (continued)				
Intervention	Type of Violence	Summary of Intervention	Evaluation Methods	Outcomes
TRUCE			Matched comparison analysis of intervention group vs neighboring communities in city	Decrease in overall violent incidents in the intervention area, but an increase in shooting incidents in the intervention area
One Vision One Life			Matched comparison analysis of intervention group vs neighboring communities in city	No evidence of a decrease in violence, and measures of violence actually increased in some neighborhoods exposed to the intervention
WITS Program	Bullying	Creates a responsible community with a uniform message and strategy that is encouraged in schools, the community, and at home. Incorporates community leaders as role models, including firefighters, police officers, paramedics, and university athletes to help reinforce the intervention messaging. Deputizes children as "constables" to keep their community safe.	Longitudinal studies comparing intervention schools and controls, using self-reported measures of victimization	Relational and physical victimization decreased significantly and at a faster rate for schools exposed to the intervention compared with control schools

Abbreviations: CPS, Child Protective Services; CSA, child sexual abuse; ED, emergency department.

economic factors in the reporting of child maltreatment and neglect.[7-12] The intersection of these factors with neighborhood, collective efficacy, and the availability of resources may impact our understanding of at-risk populations and any efforts to address the issues. The adaptation, implementation, and evaluation of community-based interventions to address physical abuse should, therefore, be considered within the context of implicit bias.

This concept of collective efficacy and mutual responsibility within communities has been applied to many community-based interventions during the last 3 decades. Here, we highlight 3 widely discussed interventions in the literature.

Strong Communities

Description

Strong Communities for Children is a community-based intervention developed as an operationalization of the strategy proposed by the US Advisory Board on Child Abuse and Neglect. It was implemented from 2002 to 2009 in 3 counties in South Carolina, with the goal to emphasize interactions that were already occurring "naturally in the institutions of everyday life.[13]" Strong Communities focused on the creation of a collective responsibility and reciprocal assistance between community members, aiming to create an environment where members of the broader community were comfortable in both asking for and offering help. The multiphase intervention gradually built a foundation for neighbor-to-neighbor involvement while simultaneously integrating health care facilities, schools, and community organizations. These specific "points of entry" were prioritized because they were seen as trusted sectors and settings that are already prominent in day-to-day community life. The 4 phases involved spreading the word, mobilizing the community, increasing family resources, and institutionalizing the provision of such resources.

Evaluation

Evaluation of Strong Communities revealed that more than 5000 individual volunteers, 199 businesses, 213 faith communities, and 85 voluntary organizations were successfully involved. More than 4000 families enrolled in the initiative, and several thousand additional families participated in sponsored events. Strong Communities parents reported less stress, more frequent help from others, and a greater sense of community and personal efficacy than parents from a matched comparison area. Hospital admissions for injuries sustained from maltreatment of children aged 4 and under decreased by 38% in the Strong Communities service area, compared with only a 13% decrease in the matched comparison area. Using data from Child Protective Services, the rates of founded cases of child maltreatment in the service area decreased in nearly all age groups, whereas the rates increased in all age groups in the comparison area. Overall, the evaluation of the Strong Communities intervention demonstrated an integration of community support that reduced child maltreatment. This success was attributed to a transformation of cultural norms within these communities.[13]

TRIPLE P: Positive Parenting Program

Description

Triple P has been applied as a strategy to prevent child abuse through a multilevel behavioral intervention designed to transform the ways in which caregivers respond and react to children.[14] The core of the Triple P system involves the creation of easily accessible learning environments within the community for parents to learn strategies that decrease caregiver–child conflicts. The system including 5 tiers, each with increasing intensity of intervention. Level 1 (Universal Triple P) is a social marketing and media campaign that involves the dissemination of basic techniques for addressing common child care challenges. This information is publicly accessible and aimed at building community awareness of resources, while also providing simple, specific tips. The advancing levels of Triple P involve more individualized and intensive approaches involving consultations and seminars on positive parenting. Level 5, or Enhanced Triple P, is the most intensive tier of the intervention that was developed for caregivers whose parenting roles are complicated by additional family stressors, including domestic conflict and mental health issues.[14]

Evaluation

The US Triple P System Population Trial was designed to assess the feasibility of implementation of Triple P strategies on a larger population level. The study design involved random assignment of 18 counties in the Southeastern United States to 1 of 2 conditions: the intervention group (implementation of Triple P) or the control group ("services as usual"). Prevention of child maltreatment was evaluated on 3 outcomes: substantiated child maltreatment recorded by Child Protective Services, out-of-home placements recorded by the foster care system, and emergency room or hospitalizations owing to child maltreatment injuries. Preintervention, the groups did not differ with respect to the 3 outcomes. After the intervention, the Triple P group was found to have statistically significant lower rates of all 3 outcomes when compared with the control, and the effect size of these results were large. Researchers concluded that implementing this intervention on a large population scale is feasible and effective based on 3 outcomes of child maltreatment rates.[15]

Durham Family Initiative

Description

This program was established in 2002 to identify the risk factors for child abuse, enhance the capacity of the community to provide resources, and increase the accessibility of resources. The Durham Family Initiative (DFI) is based on a universal assessment of families, the identification of risk, and appropriate referral to an integrated system of services in the community. A significant component of the DFI is Durham Connects, a postnatal home visitation program that incorporated universal home nurse visitation to all births in Durham County. The purpose of this initiative was to individually assess each family's needs and provide appropriate information and referrals to appropriate resources in the community.[16–18]

Evaluation

Durham and 5 matched comparison counties all showed downward trends in substantiation rates for Child Protective Services claims; however, the rates decreased more steeply in Durham after the initiation of the DFI. The rates of substantiated child maltreatment decreased by more than 63% in Durham versus less than 25% in comparison counties. Maltreatment-related diagnostic codes in hospital records decreased by 28.1% in Durham after the DFI, whereas in the comparison group, the rates increased by more than 9%. Overall, researchers estimate that this indicates a prevention of 486 cases of maltreatment over 5 years.[17] The DFI Implementation Report revealed that professionals' estimates of the rate of child abuse decreased by 11% in Durham but increased by 2% in the comparison county. A household survey found significant decreases in parental stress in randomly selected Durham neighborhoods when compared with households in the matched comparison areas. However, there were no significant changes in self-reported observed acts of potentially abusive interactions.[18]

A strength of the evidence for the Durham Connects newborn home visitation is the assessment with a randomized controlled trail that randomly assigned all births in the study period to receive either the intervention or services as usual. An analysis revealed that the intervention group had a statistically significant lower average of emergency care episodes than the control group. It demonstrated that the intervention group accessed more community resources and had a higher rate of positive parenting behaviors than control families. Finally, there was a significantly higher rating of home environment quality by blinded in-home observers in the intervention group.[19]

SEXUAL ABUSE PREVENTION

Historic attitudes surrounding child sexual abuse (CSA) have been rooted in the belief that it is a social issue that can be addressed through criminal justice systems and clinical interventions, both of which are to be used after abuse has been reported. As Letourneau and colleagues stated in 2014, "these approaches, while necessary, are fundamentally reactive, attempting to make the best of a bad situation. By comparison, the public health framework is fundamentally oriented toward prevention."[20]

In 2009, Finkelhor[21] provided a comprehensive discussion of the 2 primary strategies traditionally used for preventing CSA: management of sex offenders and school-based educational programs. He argues that offender management initiatives, although widely supported by the public and policymakers, show little evidence for the efficacy of prevention. Similarly, in terms of educational programs, Finkelhor states that although these programs are effective in promoting disclosure of abuse and prevention of self-blame, there is little evidence as to whether these programs actually reduce victimization. In discussing community prevention of sexual abuse, Finkelhor discusses the shortcomings of targeting potential abusers and that a more promising avenue may be bystander mobilization.[21]

Here we discuss 3 community-based interventions that have been implemented as large-scale public health approaches to prevention of CSA in communities. All 3 interventions have grown substantially since their initial pilot studies and have been used nationwide.

Circles of Safety (STOP IT NOW!)

Description
The first pilot program of Circles of Safety's Stop It Now! began in Vermont in 1992, testing the "application of public health campaign concepts to child sexual abuse prevention by working with the media with community-based organizations to reach adults in high-risk situations.[22]" Stop It Now! is based on the philosophy that individuals and communities can be effective advocates in the prevention of CSA. Different from the school-based education approach to the prevention of CSA, Stop It Now! focuses on changing societal norms as its long-term prevention strategy. Through a variety of avenues, they provide media messaging, prevention education materials, and training tools.[23] There are additional toolkits specifically targeting foster care populations, youth and collegiate athletic departments, and other key groups within youth communities.

One component of Stop It Now! is a confidential hotline that began through a telephone service, but has adapted throughout the past 25 years to include letters, email, and online chat options as well. The helpline was originally designed to reach adults who were at risk for sexually abusing children or those who were already perpetrators of sexual abuse, but has evolved as an avenue for all individuals to ask sensitive questions about both youth and adult sexual behaviors and provides a space for discussion and counseling about the next best step when abuse is suspected. Since 1995, more than 21,000 individuals have used the service.[24]

Evaluation
Circles of Safety Massachusetts implemented the training as a community responsibility model with a goal to increase the likelihood that adult bystanders would intervene

in situations of suspected CSA. Overall, data collected among program participants revealed increased knowledge, awareness, and confidence in responding to CSA.[25]

With an estimated 75% of children in foster care having had experienced sexual abuse either before or during foster care, a Circles of Safety program was developed to target this population specifically. An evaluation demonstrated that participants in the program increased their knowledge and awareness of child abuse within the foster care system. Additionally, there was evidence of changes in behavior and an increased confidence in handling sexual abuse among the adult participants.[26]

Grant and colleagues[24] conducted an analysis of the Stop It Now! helpline data in 2019, examining user demographics and a multitude of situational descriptors. Their analysis not only highlighted the success of the Stop It Now! program at reaching the target audience, but also demonstrated key populations and avenues for further prevention interventions. Importantly, even in situations when sexual abuse was discovered, 37% of hotline users reported that they were using the hotline before contacting authorities or other professionals. Highlighting the importance of targeting bystanders in community-based prevention programs, the majority of helpline users were those in bystander roles, and 70% of bystanders who used the hotline knew both the child who had been abused/is at risk for sexual abuse and the individual causing the abuse/at risk for abusing.

An important finding of the analysis was that nearly one-half of the hotline users were not sure whether the situation they were describing was in fact abuse, and thus they were also not sure about what to do next. The authors of this analysis conclude that helplines can be an important opportunity to protect at-risk children, because these situations are "ideal opportunities to provide an effective intervention to protect a child from abuse." Additionally, there was a significant number of contacts who used the helpline before reporting the abuse to authorities, which provides a clear avenue for encouraging and explaining the process of reporting to the caller. The results of this study reinforced the importance of targeting adult bystanders as key players in prevention efforts.[24]

Darkness to Light (Stewards of Children)

Description
This prevention campaign uses a social behavior change approach, which is a proven method to enable "changes at individual, community, and societal levels to improve health and overall well-being." It focuses on adults as key societal players in the prevention of CSA within individual "spheres of influence." The 4 main groups targeted by this intervention are (1) adults with political power or social influence, (2) adults in the community, (3) adults in youth-serving organizations, and (4) adults in the family. Three key areas are addressed by the campaign: prevention programming, advocacy for stakeholder engagement, and training to improve awareness and skills among adults.[27]

The key training program implemented by Darkness to Light is called Stewards of Children. The training is approved by several professional credentialing organizations for continuing education credits. Additional training programs include mandated reporter training, guidance on healthy touch/respectful interaction with children, bystander intervention, and a training to address age-appropriate conversations with children about boundaries.[28]

Evaluation
The Darkness to Light website provides a concise summary of 8 studies that have evaluated the Stewards of Children program.[29] In 1 study, the Stewards of Children

training was administered to undergraduate nursing students, and an analysis demonstrated a statistically significant increase in the knowledge of nursing students on the prevention, recognition, and responsible actions to take regarding CSA and trafficking.[30] A survey of more than 75,000 Texas educators was conducted to determine the impact of the Stewards of Children training on educators and showed more reports of previously unrecognized CSA to appropriate authorities. Overall, there was a 283% increase in reports of CSA to authorities by educators in the year after their Stewards of Children training compared with their reports in the year before training. These results were corroborated using data from the Texas Department of Family and Protective Services.[31]

Similarly, a study published in 2016 assessed the impact of Stewards of Children on the rates of reported cases of CSA in South Carolina. After the intervention, the intervention counties had a statistically significant increase in CSA allegations. A between-group comparison demonstrated a statistically significant difference between groups, with a trend of increasing allegations in the intervention group, and a trend of decreasing allegations in the comparison group. The authors cite that, although these results suggest that the training is successful at increasing reporting rates, it does not address whether or not it achieves prevention of CSA.[32]

Finally, a major strength of the Stewards program is being tested using a multi-site randomized controlled trial, to evaluate outcomes of the training. Funded by the Centers for Disease Control and Prevention, this trial assessed childcare professionals in 3 communities, with study participants who were assigned to 1 of 3 experimental condition groups: in-person training, web-based training, and a control group that received no training. Results indicated that immediately after the intervention and at the 3-month follow-up, the overall level of knowledge was significantly greater in the groups that were exposed to the educational materials. Additionally, preventative behaviors increased significantly more for the intervention groups compared with the control groups. Finally, when comparing the in-person versus online formats of training, there were no statistically significant differences in CSA knowledge or preventative behaviors.[33]

An interesting finding was that, despite a greater increase in preventive behaviors in the intervention groups, the control group also showed a significant increase in these behaviors over the study period. The researchers point to 2 possible explanations for this that add further value to the implementation of this program. First, they note that "the mere assessment of behaviors may impact behavior change," and second is the possibility of a "contamination effect" when participants in the intervention group may share information that they learned in the training with coworkers who had been randomly assigned to the control group.

The researchers concluded that this randomized, controlled trial adds strength to the Stewards of Children program because it demonstrated an improvement in knowledge, attitudes, and behaviors among professionals. They noted that both in-person and web-based modes of delivery were effective, although the equivalence between treatment and control groups may not fully support this.[33]

Enough Abuse Campaign

Description

This campaign began in 2003 with grant funding from the Centers for Disease Control and Prevention as a community mobilization effort in Massachusetts, but has since expanded to include efforts in 8 states. Enough Abuse involves comprehensive outreach materials and educational curricula for parents, children, families, organizations, schools, professionals, and communities. It provided workshops and presentations, and included collaborations with sex offender management coalitions. Additionally, the campaign has contributed to advocacy and legislative reform.[34] There are 3 well-recognized community frameworks for prevention that support the Enough Abuse campaign through a public health approach. For example, the campaign builds on strategies of the socioecological model, incorporating "a comprehensive approach to change that focuses on individuals, relationships, communities, and the larger society and culture." Another strategy used is the spectrum of prevention framework, which is designed to address issues in the settings where people live to drive changes in social norms. Finally, they use the framework for collaborative public health action in communities, which addresses systems changes through the integration of community stakeholders.[35]

Evaluation

Schober and colleagues[36] assessed Enough Abuse in Massachusetts, and found that between 1990 (before the campaign) and 2007 (the final year of the campaign's grant from the Centers for Disease Control and Prevention), substantiated reports of CSA in the state decreased by 69%. The authors indicate that Enough Abuse could have contributed to this decrease. The authors also cite a statewide assessment conducted in 2007, where it was found that 93% of survey respondents reported "adults should take responsibility for preventing CSA." This is in contrast with data from 2003, when only 69% of respondents stated that adults (rather than children) should take this responsibility.[36]

Enough Abuse also incorporates a training course for Kindergarten through grade 12 educators. A randomized trial demonstrated that teachers exposed to the intervention showed a significantly greater knowledge of the prevalence, behaviors, impacts, and responses to CSA than those in the control group who did not receive the training.[37] Although not peer reviewed, survey data from Enough Abuse participants are published on their website, and demonstrate that a majority of participants reported that the trainings helped them to identify abusive behaviors, address unhealthy sexual behaviors in children, and who to speak to if they suspect sexual abuse.[38]

YOUTH COMMUNITY VIOLENCE PREVENTION

As demonstrated by several of our examples elsewhere in this article, an integral aspect of developing a community-based response to any form of violence is the careful choice of the stakeholders who will be targeted as vital partners. But, as stated by Abt in a 2016 article, "Community violence is perhaps unique in the breadth of stakeholders who may contribute to an effective response. . . . This broad range of partners is appropriate given that community violence is a pervasive, persistent, and complex socioeconomic phenomenon.[39]" Abt points to the fields of public health and public safety as the key players, who together represent what he calls a "critical partnership" for the prevention of community violence. He illuminates the findings of recent criminology data, that demonstrates community violence to be relatively predictable, in that it is clustered in specific locations ("hot spots") and among specific individuals. Regarding the daunting task of decreasing community violence, Abt states that, "public and private institutions responding to violence lack the capacity to act everywhere, but they can collaborate where it matters most.[39]"

Abt and Winship coauthored a meta-analysis of community violence interventions. In their article, they discuss the "six elements of effectiveness" shared by the most successful interventions: specificity, proactivity, legitimacy, capacity, theory, and partnership. Their discussion includes what does not work in reducing community violence, including being overbroad, reactive, and attempting to work without adequate collaboration.[40] Another meta-analysis published in 2012 assessed youth violence prevention programs and similarly found that interventions that focus on more specific populations, rather than a universal approach, have been more effective.[41] Despite these proclamations and a favoring of the focus on high-risk individuals by Abt and others, a long and well-supported empirical tradition in public health favoring universally applied, population-level programs that seek to change the basic structures that underpin violence and poor health has pointed in other directions.[42–44] Moreover, a long history of mistakenly labeling individuals as being at high risk for violence continues to call into question these programs focusing on high-risk individuals and whether the programs themselves can build trust and ultimately function in the communities they seek to protect.[45]

In this section, we discuss 5 community violence prevention programs that have adapted and used the Cure Violence (CV) method.

Cure Violence

Description

CV was developed at the University of Illinois at Chicago and is built on the view of community violence as similar to a communicable disease that is transmissible from person to person. It aims to stop the spread of violence with a strategy that is reminiscent of how public health officials manage infectious disease epidemics. Different than criminal justice approaches to violence management, the CV model does not involve punishment, force, or threats thereof. It is based on behavioral change and adaptation of societal norms. The model targets individuals who are at the greatest risk for spreading gun violence and intervenes with an attempt to demonstrate that there are alternative means of conflict resolution. The intervention attempts to also spread these attitudes to the larger community in an effort to dismantle harmful societal norms surrounding violence.[46]

The intervention hires several key community members as staff. The first are violence interrupters (VIs), who are seen as important players owing to their ability to establish trusted relationships with high-risk youth in communities. VIs are often individuals who were formerly gang members or those who have been involved in criminal acts of violence. They are designed to be seen as credible individuals who are not perceived as outsiders or informants. The role of the VI is to learn about disputes in the community and monitor for signs of potential retaliation before they occur. VIs seek out such individuals and "talk them down" to communicate alternative conflict resolution strategies. A second group of key players are outreach workers who develop relationships with high-risk youth to provide resources and opportunities for housing, education, recreation, and employment. The program includes media messaging, outreach to tenant councils, faith-based organizations, and other community organizations. It relies on cooperation with local law enforcement to understand crime patterns and to assist in the recruitment of VIs and outreach workers within communities.[46]

Evaluation

CV has been adapted and implemented in several cities, with corresponding evaluations of the program impact. In summary, all of these evaluations show mixed support for the success of the CV model, and owing to these results, the US Department of Justice Crime Solutions database categorizes the CV program as "promising."[47] As described by Butts and colleagues,[46] evaluations of complex interventions for community violence prevention are extremely challenging. There are innumerable confounding factors (both positive and negative) that contribute to violent acts and community violence trends that are independent of the direct effects attributable to intervention efforts. Ideally, the strongest evidence for an intervention comes from a randomized controlled trial. Butts and colleagues[46] discuss that this would require a much larger number of neighborhoods for an extended period of time to adequately and reliably monitor change. Here, we briefly discuss the implementation and evaluation of CV in 5 US cities.

Cure violence in Chicago: CeaseFire

With funding from the US Department of Justice, the first comprehensive study of the CV method was based on a program called CeaseFire that was implemented in several neighborhoods in Chicago.[48] Overall, the evaluation found that, after the implementation of the CV program, there was a significant decrease in all shots reported in 4 of the 7 neighborhoods included in the analysis. The researchers described that in 4 communities, the decrease in size and intensity of shooting "hot spots" were attributable to the introduction of CeaseFire, with these communities overall outperforming matched comparison sites with respect to violence.

A gang homicide network analysis found that, in some sites, there were improvements in gang involvement in homicide, retaliatory killing, and violence density when compared with the matched comparison areas. However, this finding was not consistent across sites and there were wide variations in sites on the gang-related outcomes. Despite the mixed results of violent crime data, a survey of program participants did indicate that the program succeeded in reaching its target population.

The evaluation report also demonstrated several key points that highlight the difficulty in analyzing this type of intervention. A particularly salient example was related to the impact of VIs. The results point to the success of VIs in diffusing the conflicts that often lead to retaliatory violence. However, there was evidence that the impact of VIs crossed geographic boundaries, with collaborations in neighboring communities as well. Although this spillover effect is a positive impact of the program, it explains a difficulty in the evaluation of data from sharply defined geographic areas: both gang activities and the positive impact of VIs do not organically adhere to sharply defined regions. As the evaluation report explains, the positive impact of the intervention could have affected the matched comparison areas within the city and also could have masked the positive outcomes within the targeted neighborhoods.[48]

Cure violence in Baltimore: safe streets

CV was implemented in Baltimore as the SafeStreets program. Similar to what was discovered in Chicago, the effects of the program extended to neighborhoods that bordered the targeted areas. An important strength of the evaluation of Baltimore's program was that it incorporated analysis of the program impact on these neighboring spillover areas as well. Overall, it was concluded that across all sites and their neighboring areas, the impact of SafeStreets is estimated to equate to 5.4 fewer homicide incidents (2.8 in intervention areas, 2.6 in border areas) and 34.6 fewer nonfatal shooting incidents (17.1 in intervention areas and 17.5 in border areas).[49]

Again, these authors cited difficulties in selecting appropriate comparison areas. Additionally, there was one neighborhood that actually experienced an increase in homicides after the SafeStreets implementation. However, researchers do not believe this increase was attributable to the program activities, but rather the conditions in the community that prompted the initiation of the program in the first place. The evaluators concluded that, despite mixed results in program impact, 3 of the 4 neighborhoods targeted by the intervention experienced statistically significant "relatively large program-related reductions in at least one measure of gun violence without also having a statistically significant increase in another measure of gun violence."[49] Nearly 90% of participants reported that outreach workers assisted them in finding a job, and 95% reported they were assisted in getting into a school or a GED program. These outreach workers helped more than one-half of the participants settle disputes (28% of which involved guns). The engagement of hundreds of high-risk youth led to the mediation of 200 disputes that had the potential to lead to a shooting.[50]

Cure violence in Brooklyn: Save Our Streets
CV was implemented in Brooklyn, New York, as Save Our Streets. Overall, the evaluation revealed that the average shooting rates decreased by 6% in the implementation neighborhood, whereas they increased by 18% to 28% in matched comparison areas. The difference between the intervention neighborhoods was statistically significant, and translates into an estimate that gun violence in the intervention area was 20% lower than what it would have been without the intervention, if trends would have mirrored the adjacent matched areas.[51]

Cure violence in Phoenix: TRUCE
The TRUCE program, an adaptation of CV in Phoenix, Arizona, was associated with a significant decrease in overall violent incidents (16 fewer incidents on average per month); however, this decrease was mostly driven by a decrease in assaults. In fact, there was a significant increase of 3.2 shootings on average per month, controlling for matched comparison areas. Additionally, implementation success was partly hindered by a lack of involvement of local faith-based community organizations.[52]

Cure violence in Pittsburgh: One Vision One Life
CV was implemented in Pittsburgh as One Vision One Life, albeit with some changes to the originally developed model. Evaluation did not reveal quantitative evidence that the program decreased violence, including homicide rates, aggravated assaults, and gun assaults. Additionally, there was evidence that these measures even increased in some areas during the intervention periods. Further, there was no associated change in homicide in the spillover areas, as demonstrated in other cities.[53]

COMMUNITY-BASED BULLYING PREVENTION

Bullying prevention has traditionally focused on school-based approaches; however, Holt and colleagues[54] discuss the socioecological framework as a promising model for addressing bullying prevention in a community-based effort. The authors cite 3 specific resources that are available in almost all communities, namely, heath care, extracurricular programs, and law enforcement, as key spheres for the implementation of antibullying campaigns.[54] Here we discuss a program that incorporates these community resources into the prevention of peer violence or bullying.

WITS Program

Description
WITS is a group of programs developed in Canada as an effort to integrate schools, families, and communities to decrease and prevent peer victimization. The overall goal of the program is to build a responsive community by engaging teachers, parents, school counselors, older students, community leaders, and emergency services personnel. It implements a common language and strategy within a broad array of

children's social networks. Adults and older youth within the community are taught this common language to assist young children in "using their WITS" to avoid peer aggression. WITS is an acronym that stands for Walk away, Ignore the bully, Talk it out, and Seek Help. Essentially this acronym is created as a code word that will ideally be uniformly used within schools, families, and the surrounding community, creating consistency in children's environments, such that children "learn that conflicts are resolvable and that adults know how to help them." This is a multisetting approach that incorporates community leaders into the implementation of this program. Police, firefighters, and paramedics serve as liaisons, and after completing a training module, these leaders conduct a swearing in ceremony, where children from Kindergarten to third grade are "deputized as WITS special constables" who promise to keep their school and community a safe place. These emergency services personnel are joined by other community role models, including university and high school athletes, all of whom make school visits throughout the year to further reinforce the message of the intervention. Siblings, friends, parents, and caregivers are provided with multimedia tools to assist them in incorporating the WITS program at home.[55,56]

Evaluation

A longitudinal study was conducted to evaluate 11 WITS program schools, comparing them with 6 control schools. The evaluation revealed that classroom levels of both relational victimization and physical victimization decreased significantly in schools that received the WITS intervention, compared with the control schools that had similar levels of school poverty.[57] A second longitudinal study included 6 program schools and 5 control schools. The major findings were that the rate of decline for both physical and relational victimization was significantly greater in WITS program schools compared with control schools.[58]

SUMMARY

Decreasing violence against children has traditionally been reactive in nature and focused on the punishment of perpetrators after abuse occurs. More recently, community-based interventions have been developed as a preventive approach. These interventions are based on the evidence that the surrounding environment can expose individuals to factors that make them more or less susceptible to violence. Furthermore, there are key stakeholders within the community who can be mobilized effectively to mediate such factors, particularly when there is a collective efficacy. Like all community-based initiatives, such programs face many challenges, especially related to outcomes evaluation and the potential to mislabel and enroll individuals as high risk when they are not. Evaluation with randomized controlled trials is often not feasible in assessing the outcomes of community-based programs, although programs that have been evaluated using trials can be better positioned for success. Additionally, evaluation does not simply assess the effectiveness of an intervention, but the effectiveness of it within a specific community context. This type of program requires long-term funding, which is often a barrier to continued implementation and successful recognition. And, as stated by an Institute of Medicine committee, "the costs of these programs are immediate, but the benefits are often deferred to the future."[1]

Despite the challenges faced in the implementation and evaluation of these programs, there have been measurable successes in the prevention of violence against children through community-engaged approaches. A multitude of resources are available that can guide communities in choosing an intervention that can be adapted to target specific problems within their own local context.

CLINICS CARE POINTS

- Large disparities exist between different communities and their rates of violence against children.
- Results of meta-analyses demonstrate that the strongest predictors of child maltreatment and sexual abuse are related to poverty, unemployment, and lack of neighborhood collective efficacy and social networks.
- Violence against children has been increasingly exposed as a public health crisis within the past 30 years.
- Community-based interventions to prevent violence are similar to other public health approaches in that they target a broad range of settings and sectors and emphasize collaboration.
- Bystander mobilization is a shared feature of many community-based violence prevention programs and focuses on prioritizing adults in the prevention of violence against children rather than targeting children themselves.
- The evaluation of community-based interventions is challenging owing to the length of time required to see an impact, an obscured cost–benefit relationship, and the limited feasibility of conducting randomized controlled trials.
- Securing and maintaining funding for community-based interventions is an additional barrier owing to the large upfront costs and the length of time needed to ascertain an impact

DISCLOSURE

The authors have nothing to disclose.

REFERENCES

1. Committee on Valuing Community-Based, Non-Clinical Prevention Programs. Board on population health and public health practice; institute of medicine. an integrated framework for assessing the value of community-based prevention. Washington (DC): National Academies Press (US); 2012. Available at: https://www.ncbi.nlm.nih.gov/books/NBK20692 doi:10.17226/13487.
2. U.S. Department of Health and Human Services, U.S. Advisory board on child abuse and neglect. neighbors helping neighbors: a new national strategy for the protection of children. Washington, DC: U.S. Government Printing Office; 1993.
3. Garbarino J, Sherman D. High-risk neighborhoods and high-risk families: the human ecology of child maltreatment. Child Development 1980;51(1):188–98.
4. Coulton CJ, Korbin JE, Su M, et al. Community level factors and child maltreatment rates. Child Development 1995;66(5):1262–76.
5. Molnar BE, Goerge RM, Gilsanz P, et al. Neighborhood-level social processes and substantiated cases of child maltreatment. Child Abuse Negl 2016;51:41–53.
6. Drake B, Pandey S. Understanding the relationship between neighborhood poverty and specific types of child maltreatment. Child Abuse Negl 1996;20(11):1003–18.
7. Rojas M, Walker-Descartes I, Laraque-Arena D. An experimental study of implicit racial bias in recognition of child abuse. Am J Health Behav 2017;41(3):358–67.
8. Lane WG, Roubin DM, Monteith R, et al. Racial differences in the evaluation of pediatric fractures for physical abuse. JAMA 2002;288(13):1603–9.

9. Laskey AL, Stump TE, Perkins SM, et al. Influence of race and socioeconomic status on the diagnosis of child abuse: a randomized study. J Pediatr 2012; 160:1003–8.
10. Wood JN, Hall M, Schilling S, et al. Disparities in the evaluation and diagnosis of abuse among infants with traumatic brain injury. Pediatrics 2010;126(3):408–14.
11. Flaherty EG, Sege RD, Griffith J, et al. From suspicion of physical child abuse to reporting: primary care clinician decision-making. Pediatrics 2008;122(3):611–9.
12. Jenny C, Hymel KP, Ritzen A, et al. Analysis of missed cases of abusive head trauma. JAMA 1999;282(7):621–9.
13. Melton GB, McLeigh JD. The nature, logic, and significance of strong communities for children. Int J Child Malt 2020;3:125–61.
14. Sanders MR, Turner KM, Markie-Dadds C. The development and dissemination of the Triple P-positive parenting program: a multilevel, evidence-based system of parenting and family support. Prev Sci 2002;3(3):173–89.
15. Prinz RJ, Sanders MR, Shapiro CJ, et al. Population-based prevention of child maltreatment: the U.S. Triple p system population trial [published correction appears in Prev Sci. 2015 Jan;16(1):168]. Prev Sci 2009;10(1):1–12.
16. Dodge KA, Berlin LJ, Epstein M, et al. The Durham Family Initiative: a preventive system of care. Child Welfare 2004;83(2):109–28.
17. Rosanbalm KD, Dodge KA, Murphy R, et al. Evaluation of a collaborative community-based child maltreatment prevention initiative. Prot Child 2010; 25(4):8–23.
18. Daro D, Huang L, English B. The duke endowment child abuse prevention initiative: Durham Family Initiative implementation report. Chicago (IL): Chapin Hall at the University of Chicago; 2009.
19. Dodge KA, Goodman WB, Murphy RA, et al. Implementation and randomized controlled trial evaluation of universal postnatal nurse home visiting. Am J Public Health 2014;104(Suppl 1):S136–43.
20. Letourneau EJ, Eaton WW, Bass J, et al. The need for a comprehensive public health approach to preventing child sexual abuse. Public Health Rep 2014; 129(3):222–8.
21. Finkelhor D. The prevention of childhood sexual abuse. Future Child 2009;19(2): 169–94.
22. Stop it now! Vermont: brief history. Available at: https://www.stopitnow.org/our-work/about-us/prevention-advocacy/stop-it-now-vermont. Accessed August 29, 2020.
23. Stop it now! Vermont: our approach. Available at: https://www.stopitnow.org/about-us/our-approach. Accessed August 29, 2020.
24. Grant B, Shields R, Tabachnick J, et al. "I didn't know where to go": an examination of stop it now!'s sexual abuse prevention helpline. J Interpers Violence 2019; 34(20):4225–53.
25. Evaluation of stop it now's circles of safety program. 2018. Available at: https://www.stopitnow.org/sites/default/files/documents/files/executive_summary_final.pdf. Accessed August 29, 2020.
26. Evaluation of the Circles of Safety for Foster Care program. 2017. Available at: https://www.stopitnow.org/sites/default/files/documents/files/final_evaluation.pdf. Accessed August 29, 2020.
27. Darkness to light: our approach. Available at: https://www.d2l.org/our-work/our-approach/. Accessed August 29, 2020.
28. Darkness to light: the training. Available at: https://www.d2l.org/education/the-training/. Accessed August 29, 2020.

29. Stewards of children—evidence-based prevention training. Available at: https://www.d2l.org/our-work/research/. Accessed August 29, 2020.

30. Taylor LE, Harris HS. Stewards of children education: increasing undergraduate nursing student knowledge of child sexual abuse. Nurse Educ Today 2018;60:147–50.

31. Townsend C, Haviland M. The impact of child sexual abuse training for educators on reporting and victim outcomes: the Texas Educator Initiative. 2016. Charleston, S.C., Darkness to Light. Available at: https://www.d2l.org/wp-content/uploads/2017/03/The-Impact-of-CSA-Training-for-Educators.pdf. Accessed August 29, 2020.

32. Letourneau EJ, Nietert PJ, Rheingold AA. Initial assessment of stewards of children program effects on child sexual abuse reporting rates in selected South Carolina counties. Child Maltreat 2016;21(1):74–9.

33. Rheingold AA, Zajac K, Chapman JE, et al. Child sexual abuse prevention training for childcare professionals: an independent multi-site randomized controlled trial of Stewards of Children. Prev Sci 2015;16(3):374–85.

34. The enough abuse campaign: history. Available at: https://www.enoughabuse.org/the-campaign/history.html. Accessed August 29, 2020.

35. The enough abuse campaign: enough abuse frameworks for prevention. Available at: https://www.enoughabuse.org/the-campaign/stragegies-and-results.html. Accessed August 29, 2020.

36. Schober DJ, Fawcett SB, Bernier J. The enough abuse campaign: building the movement to prevent child sexual abuse in Massachusetts. J Child Sex Abus 2012;21(4):456–69.

37. Gushwa M, Bernier J, Robinson D. Advancing child sexual abuse prevention in schools: an exploration of the effectiveness of the enough! online training program for K-12 teachers. J Child Sex Abus 2019;28(2):144–59.

38. The enough abuse campaign: effectiveness. Available at: https://www.enoughabuse.org/the-campaign/results.html. Accessed August 29, 2020.

39. Abt TP. Towards a framework for preventing community violence among youth. Psychol Health Med 2017;22(sup1):266–85.

40. Abt TP, Winship C. "What works" in reducing community violence: a meta-review and field study for the northern triangle. Washington, DC: United States Agency for International Development; 2016.

41. Matjasko JL, Vivolo-Kantor AM, Massetti GM, et al. A systematic meta-review of evaluations of youth violence prevention programs: common and divergent findings from 25 years of meta-analyses and systematic reviews. Aggress Violent Behav 2012;17(6):540–52.

42. Rose G. Sick individuals and sick populations. Int J Epidemiol 2001;30(3):427–32.

43. Frieden TR. A framework for public health action: the health impact pyramid. Am J Public Health 2010;100(4):590–5.

44. Branas CC, MacDonald JM. A simple strategy to transform health, all over the place. J Public Health Manag Pract 2014;20(2):157.

45. Available at: https://www.nytimes.com/2018/03/23/opinion/superpredator-myth.html. Accessed August 29, 2020.

46. Butts JA, Roman CG, Bostwick L, et al. Cure Violence: a public health model to reduce gun violence. Annu Rev Public Health 2015;36:39–53.

47. Program profile: Cure Violence. the national institute of justice: crime solutions. 2011. Available at: https://crimesolutions.ojp.gov/programdetails?id=205&ID=205. Accessed August 29, 2020.

48. Skogan WG, Hartnett SM, Bump N, et al. Evaluation of CeaseFire-Chicago. Evanston (IL): Northwestern University; 2008; 2009.
49. Webster DW, Whitehill JM, Vernick JS, et al. Effects of Baltimore's Safe Streets program on gun violence: a replication of Chicago's Ceasefire Program. J Urban Health 2013;90(1):27–40.
50. Webster DW, Mendel Whitehill J, Vernick JS, et al. Evaluation of Baltimore's Safe Streets program: effects on attitudes, participants' experiences, and Gun Violence. Baltimore (MD): Johns Hopkins Cent. Prev. Youth Violence; 2012.
51. Picard-Fritsche S, Cerniglia L. Testing a public health approach to gun violence: an evaluation of crown heights save our streets, a replication of the Cure Violence model. New York: Cent Court Innov; 2013.
52. Fox AM, Katz CM, Choate DE, et al. Evaluation of the Phoenix TRUCE project: a replication of Chicago CeaseFire. Justice Q 2015;32:85–115.
53. Wilson JM, Chermak S. Community-driven violence reduction programs: examining Pittsburgh's One Vision One Life. Criminol Public Policy 2011;10:993–1027.
54. Holt MK, Raczynski K, Frey KS, et al. School and community-based approaches for preventing bullying. J Sch Violence 2013;12(3):238–52.
55. The WITS programs foundation: WITS primary program. Available at: https://witsprogram.ca/school/wits-primary-program/. Accessed August 29, 2020.
56. Leadbeater B, Hoglund W. Changing the social contexts of peer victimization. J Can Acad Child Adolesc Psychiatry 2006;15(1):21–6.
57. Leadbeater B, Hoglund W, Woods T. Changing contexts? The effects of a primary prevention program on classroom levels of peer relational and physical victimization. J Community Psychol 2003;31(4):397–418.
58. Leadbeater B, Sukhawathanakul P. Multicomponent programs for reducing peer victimization in early elementary school: a longitudinal evaluation of the WITS Primary Program. J Community Psychol 2011;39:606–20.

Moving?

Make sure your subscription moves with you!

To notify us of your new address, find your **Clinics Account Number** (located on your mailing label above your name), and contact customer service at:

Email: **journalscustomerservice-usa@elsevier.com**

800-654-2452 (subscribers in the U.S. & Canada)
314-447-8871 (subscribers outside of the U.S. & Canada)

Fax number: **314-447-8029**

Elsevier Health Sciences Division
Subscription Customer Service
3251 Riverport Lane
Maryland Heights, MO 63043

*To ensure uninterrupted delivery of your subscription, please notify us at least 4 weeks in advance of move.

Sheridan
Hanover, PA USA
August 29, 2023